Proven Natural Ways to

Lower

I0210260

High Blood Pressure

30 Proven Natural Superfoods To Control & Lower Your High Blood Pressure

By *Louise Jiannes*

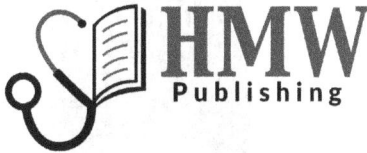

For more great books visit:

HMWPublishing.com

Download another book for

Free

I want to thank you for purchasing this book and offer you another book (just as long and valuable as this book), "Health & Fitness Mistakes You Don't Know You're Making", completely free.

Visit the link below to signup and receive it:

www.hmwpublishing.com/gift

In this book, I will break down the most common health & fitness mistakes, you are probably committing right now, and I will reveal how you can easily get in the best shape of your life!

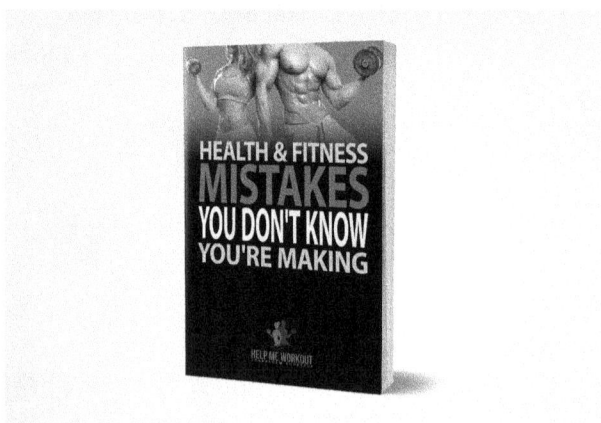

In addition to this valuable gift, you will also have an opportunity to get our new books for free, enter giveaways, and receive other valuable emails from me. Again, visit the link to sign up:

www.hmwpublishing.com/gift

TABLE OF CONTENT

INTRODUCTION

The rising number of people affected by high blood pressure had brought awareness to the public but being aware of the sickness or its presence is not enough to exclude you from its deadly fang.

For decades, this sickness had been ignored and overlooked because of its silent symptoms which earned it the title of being the "Silent Killer" but as government's efforts are driven towards minimizing if not eliminating its presence; attention to this illness is being brought forward to the public.

If you are one of the many people, who are not comfortable living with the idea that you could be affected by this illness without actually knowing it. This book, *"Proven Natural Ways to Lower High Blood Pressure"* will equip you with the knowledge of high blood pressure and how to reverse it naturally without the use of medications.

Furthermore, while we are discussing the treatment of high blood pressure, we should also be aware of its preventive measures. Know all the essential facts about this silent killer to live a healthier life!

Also, before you get started, I recommend you **joining our email newsletter** to receive updates on any upcoming new book releases or promotions. You can sign-up for free, and as a bonus, you will receive a free gift. Our *"Health & Fitness Mistakes You Don't Know You're Making"* book! This book has been written to demystify, expose the top do's and don'ts and to finally equip you with the information you need to get in the best shape of your life. Due to the overwhelming amount of mis-information and lies told by magazines and self-proclaimed "gurus", it's becoming harder and harder to get reliable information to get in shape. As opposed to having to go through dozens of biased, unreliable and un-trustworthy sources to get your health & fitness information. Everything you need to help you has been broken down in this book for you to easily follow and to immediately get results to achieve your desired fitness goals in the shortest amount of time.

Once again, to join our free email newsletter and to receive a free copy of this valuable book, please visit the link and signup now:

www.hmwpublishing.com/gift

CHAPTER 1 – OVERVIEW ON HIGH BLOOD PRESSURE

High blood pressure is one of the primary contributing causes of death in the United States. According to the recent report released by the Center for Disease and Control Prevention, about 75 million American adults have high blood pressure. To give you a quick calculation, that's one out of every three adult Americans or around 29% of the American population. Approximately $46 billion is spent by the nation each year to cover health care services and medications. This also includes missed days of work due to hypertension.

Symptoms of high blood pressure are sometimes so mild that it's hard to detect. However, its results can be deadly and therefore must be taken with the utmost concern. Untreated, high blood pressure, also known as "hypertension can damage and can leave scars to the arteries which can also be found even in people who are normally calm and relaxed. The "Silent Killer," as it carries no initial symptoms, is a long-term illness, which can eventually lead to complications and death.

HOW CAN HIGH BLOOD PRESSURE OCCUR?

High blood pressure is the impact of the blood created against the wall of the arteries as it circulates inside the human body. The blood pressure is determined by the amount of blood pumped by the heart against its resistance as it flows through the arteries.

When there are some blockades like cholesterol build up, scarring or plaque in the arteries, it affects the elasticity of the arterial walls and narrows the way of the bloodstream, thereby creating more pressure as the heart pumps harder to get the blood through so that it can reach the different parts of the body. Such increase in pressure can damage the muscles and valves of the heart and may result in heart failure. Damages to the vessels supplying blood and oxygen to kidneys and brain eventually create a negative impact on these body organs.

Too much pressure in the blood vessels and arterial walls can cause serious problems. Healthy arteries are usually semi-flexible tissues and muscles that are fine, smooth, elastic and stretchable, so blood flows smoothly through them when the heart starts to pump mildly. However, when there are blockades, the heart is forced to pump more thereby stretching the walls of the arteries, and if done too much, it could break the lining of the arterial walling. Once blood vessels are broken, it could lead to stroke, kidneys malfunction, peripheral vascular failure or heart attack, which causes death to the majority of its victims.

It is, therefore, essential to keep your blood pressure at a level to reduce the risk of blood vessels from getting overstretch beyond its limit. Uncontrolled blood pressure increases the risk of more serious health or medical problems to occur.

Chapter 2: The Dangers of Having High Blood Pressure

High blood pressure is steadily increasing in modern societies due to an unhealthy lifestyle. This can be very disturbing if you are not fully aware of its implications in your health condition, but if you do, you can look for useful options to reverse its effects.

High blood pressure can silently do some serious damage to your body system long before the onset of symptoms. Taking it for granted can result to a disability, a life of suffering, and even a severe heart attack. People who are left untreated of high blood pressure die of ischemic heart disease or reduced blood flow. Others die of stroke. A shift in lifestyle and treatment can help control your high blood pressure to reduce these life-threatening risks. Now, let's take a look to some of the damages it can cause to your body.

DAMAGE TO YOUR ARTERIES

When your arteries are healthy, they are flexible, elastic, and strong with a smooth inner lining along the walls to let the blood flow freely as it circulates the body. This is a vital process as it supplies nutrients and oxygen to vital tissues and organs. When the bloodstream is clogged, it causes an increase in pressure in the arterial wall as the heart pumps vigorously to let the blood flow in. As a result, you could be experiencing the following:

- *DAMAGED AND NARROWED ARTERIES*

  When you have an unhealthy lifestyle, your body can collect fats from your diet and store them in your arteries, clogging the flow of the bloodstream and your artery walls become less elastic. This limits the flow of blood in your body.

- *ANEURYSM*

  Eventually, the constant pressure of blood against the weakened artery lining may cause a part of the wall to form a bulge. This condition is called "an aneurysm." An aneurysm can rupture anytime and can cause internal bleeding in any of your arteries, but mostly it occurs in the aorta or the largest artery in your body.

DAMAGE TO THE HEART

Since your heart pumps blood to your body, uncontrolled high blood pressure can do damage to your heart in many ways.

- *CORONARY ARTERY DISEASE*

  This condition affects the arteries that supply blood to the body. The disease narrows down the arteries and limits the blood to flow freely through the arteries. When you have this illness, you can experience irregular heart rhythms known as (arrhythmias), chest pains or an irregular heart attack.

- *ENLARGED LEFT HEART*

  When your heart is forced to exert vigorously to pump blood into your body, it causes the left ventricle to become stiffen or thickens (left ventricular hypertrophy). These changes also limit the ventricle's ability to pump blood thereby increasing the risk of a heart failure, heart, attack and sudden cardiac death.

- *HEART FAILURE*

  Eventually, the strain on your heart caused by the high blood pressure weakens your heart muscles and makes them work less efficiently. If this continues to go on, this condition will just wear out your heart. Your heart will wear out in time and fail and if there's some damage caused by heart attack, they add more to the existing problem.

DAMAGE TO THE BRAIN

Like your heart, the brain depends on the supply of blood to nourish it so it can work properly to survive. However, when there is high blood pressure, it can cause problems including what we have here below.

- *TRANSIENT ISCHEMIC ATTACK (TIA)*

  Considered as a "mini-stroke," this condition is a temporary disruption of the blood supply to your brain. Transient Ischemic Condition is often caused by atherosclerosis or a blood clot. Both of these can arise when there is high blood pressure, and the presence of the TIA is a warning that you're at risk for a full-blown stroke.

* *STROKE*

  When part of your brain is deprived of oxygen and nutrients supplied by your blood vessels, it will cause the death of your brain cells. So, when you have high blood pressure that is left uncontrolled or neglected, this can cause the narrowing, rupture or leaks in your blood vessels leading to the brain. High blood pressure can likewise cause blood clotting in the arteries blocking the blood flow to your brain and causing a stroke.

- *DEMENTIA*

  This condition is associated with problems in cognitive abilities – thinking, speaking, reasoning, memory, vision, and movements. There are various causes of dementia including vascular dementia, which is attained through narrowing and blockage of the arteries that supply blood to the brain. It can also result in a stroke that causes an interruption in the blood flow leading to the brain. In any of these cases, it's the high blood pressure that mainly causes it.

- *MILD COGNITIVE IMPAIRMENT*

  There is a transition stage, which occurs between the changes in understanding, and memory as one grows old and the more severe problems develop when one gets, for example, an Alzheimer's disease. Like dementia, this results from blocked blood flow when high blood pressure damages arteries.

DAMAGE TO YOUR KIDNEYS

Typically, it's the function of your kidneys to filter excess waste and fluids from your blood, though this process depends on your healthy blood vessels. When high blood pressure injures your blood vessels leading to your kidneys, it may cause numerous types of kidney diseases (nephropathy). If you have diabetes, this can even worsen the damage.

• *KIDNEY FAILURE*

Kidney failure is caused by high blood pressure as it brings damage both to the large arteries leading to your kidneys and the tiny blood vessels (glomeruli) within the kidneys. Damage to either of these two affects the normal function of your kidneys hindering it from efficiently filtering waste from the blood. In the end, a dangerous level of waste and fluids can accumulate in your body and may ultimately require dialysis or a kidney transplant.

- *KIDNEY SCARRING*

  Glomerulosclerosis is a type of kidney damage caused by scarring of the glomeruli (glue-MER-u-li). The glomeruli are tiny clusters of blood vessels within your kidneys that filter fluid and waste from your blood. Glomerulosclerosis can leave your kidneys unable to filter waste efficiently, leading to kidney failure.

- *KIDNEY ARTERY ANEURYSM*

  This is a type of an aneurysm leading to the kidney. One potential cause of this disease is atherosclerosis, which damages and weakens the artery wall. In the long run, a weakened artery can cause a section to form an aneurysm, which can rupture anytime and cause a life threatening internal bleeding.

CHAPTER 3: CAUSES AND SYMPTOMS

It's not easy to identify the exact cause of high blood pressure, but numerous factors and conditions that may somehow have contributed to its development.

Here are some among them:

- Obesity or overweight

- Lack of physical activity

- Too much consumption of salt and alcohol

- Smoking

- Genes and family history including high blood pressure

- Unmanageable stress

- Chronic kidney ailments

- Thyroid and adrenal disorders

- Sleep apnea

ESSENTIAL HYPERTENSION

In the United States, more than 95% of reported high blood pressure cases, the underlying cause is not determined. For this type of high blood pressure, people in the medical world call it as the "essential hypertension."

Mysterious as it is, essential hypertension has been linked to specific risk factors. High blood pressure tends to affect more males than their female counterparts and is likewise observed to run in the family.

Moreover, age and race also play a vital role. African Americans living in the United States are twice as more likely to have high blood pressure compared to Caucasians, but the gap decreases at around age 44. Many black women have the highest reported incidence of high blood pressure at the age of 65 and above.

Other factors that affect essential hypertension are diet and lifestyle. The link between salt and high blood pressure has long been established. Japanese people living in the northern islands of Japan are known to consume more salt per capita than people in the rest of the world, and they've got the highest incidence of essential hypertension. Conversationally, who don't use salt to their food have no traces of essential hypertension.

People with high blood pressure are hypersensitive, in other words, this means that even a small excess of salt added to what is typically needed by the body can send their blood pressure to soar up. Other factors that count in the presence of essential high blood pressure are an insufficiency in calcium, magnesium, and potassium, chronic alcohol consumption, obesity, and diabetes.

SECONDARY HYPERTENSION

Contrary to essential high blood pressure is the Secondary High Blood Pressure or "secondary hypertension." This type of high blood pressure, the direct cause is somehow pinpointed, and kidney disease ranks the highest among the many causes of secondary hypertension.

This type of high blood pressure can be triggered by tumors and other abnormalities, which cause the adrenal glands to produce excess amounts of hormones that elevate the blood pressure.

The factors that can send blood pressure to rise include:

- Pregnancy

- Birth control pills particularly those that contain estrogen

- Drugs that constrict blood vessels

Chapter 4: Preventive Measures for High Blood Pressures

Making an extra effort to prevent the onset of high blood pressure can help in the reduction of stroke, heart attack, and many other serious illnesses that can lead to death. If you are at risk for high blood pressure, it's best for you to take these preventive measures.

Preventive Factors You Can Control

Some factors like, age and genes including family medical histories are elements that are beyond your control. Therefore, if you want to prevent the onset of high blood pressure, you need to focus on the risk factors that you can change. We are not able to do something about our age or what constitutes our

DNA, but we can always change our lifestyle for a better and healthy one.

Here are some ways to consider in shifting to a healthy lifestyle.

• *MAINTAIN A NORMAL AND HEALTHY WEIGHT*

Maintaining a healthy weight is crucial when it comes to hypertension. Overweight and obesity can lead to more complications, which can eventually lead to death. People who are overweight need to lose weight and if you are of average weight, then avoid adding more pounds. Finally, if you are carrying extra weight, lose as much as ten pounds to help prevent the occurrence of high blood pressure. There are online resources to help you know your ideal weight and your body mass index (BMI).

- *EAT A BALANCED DIET*

  Eating a healthy balanced diet can help keep your blood pressure under control. Eat foods that are rich in potassium while keeping a limit on calories, fat, sodium, and sugar. DASH Diet is known to help in managing high blood pressure.

- *CUT BACK SODIUM CONSUMPTION*

  The higher the sodium intake you have, the higher the blood pressure rises. Therefore, it is better to cut down on your sodium intake by avoiding foods that are high in sodium content like packaged foods and processed food. It may also help to prevent adding salt to your meals.

- *LIMIT ALCOHOL INTAKE*

  Drinking too much alcohol thickens the blood and therefore creates more pressure for the heart to have it flowed smoothly and freely. Thus, avoid having more than a drink in a day.

- *HAVE A REGULAR EXERCISE*

It takes activity to make one healthy, and physical activity is crucial when referring to high blood pressure. The more exercise you have, the better. However, even a little bit of exercise can do so much to lessen the risk of hypertension. Start doing a moderate amount of exercise for about 30 minutes. Starting by training two to three times a week is an ideal target to begin.

- *MONITOR YOUR BLOOD PRESSURE*

  After you have done with the ways stated above, make sure that you regularly monitor your blood pressure. To do this, you can either go to a clinic or do this at home. Since hypertension often shows no apparent symptoms, only the blood pressure reading can give you a definite measurement of your blood pressure. Blood pressure reading in the range of 120-139/80-89 millimeters of mercury (mmHg) puts you at an increased risk of developing high blood pressure.

- *CHANGING YOUR BAD HABITS*

  Finally, take a look at your lifestyle and see what among your habits needs to change. Try conquering small goals like eating fruits and vegetables instead of junk foods in between meals. Make these habits as part of your daily routine.

CHAPTER 5: PROVEN WAYS TO CONTROL HIGH BLOOD PRESSURE WITHOUT MEDICATION

Although we have introduced some preventive measures to get away from having high blood pressure, still we know it is not that easy to make a 360 degrees shift in your lifestyle. With the kind of modern life we have today, when almost everyone is always on the go, we fill in our stomachs with ready-to-eat foods right out of the package. We know that these foods are far from being healthy and unless you are determined to change your ways, you need to refrain from eating theses kind of foods.

WHAT ABOUT IF YOU ALREADY HAVE THAT SICKNESS IN YOU?

As I have stated, high blood pressure is a sickness that must not be ignored. Deaths related to high blood pressure run to almost 100,000 each year and is still rapidly increasing. Some people just ignore their problem while others choose medications with harmful effects. But, nowadays, the majority of people resort back to the use of simple natural remedies to treat high blood pressure. There are many natural remedies proven over the years to combat high blood pressure.

Before considering drug medication for your hypertension problem, take note of the following facts:

✓ Pharmaceutical companies are considered to be one of the most lucrative businesses in the 21st Century.

✓ The number of hospitals has grown these past decades exponentially. Before it was believed to be due to baby boomers or those in their retirement age, however, recent studies are showing that people tend to rely more on doctors nowadays for every aspect of their physical health.

✓ Insurance rates and coverage have grown too high partly due to inflated medical and prescriptions cost.

Obviously, not all drugs are dangerous. Many have their purpose in life are beneficial to our society. However, some drugs are harmful in some ways as they are harsh and carry deadly side effects in many ways.

Nonetheless, millions of people are still choosing to forego using medications with dangerous side effects and instead resort to the holistic and natural treatment of high blood pressure. With holistic treatment, we refer to the kind of healing that view the wholeness of a person. That is, instead of focusing on the treatment of a disease, the holistic approach looks at an individual's overall physical, emotional, mental, and spiritual well being before recommending treatment.

This holistic approach to natural treatment might involve a nutritional diet, regular exercise, meditation, and much more. Attacking high blood pressure on many different angles can completely cure the person without the use of drug medication!

HOW CAN ONE BENEFIT FROM THE NATURAL TREATMENT?

Beside from the avoidance of the life-threatening side effects of drugs, there are various reasons why you need to consider treating high blood pressure naturally.

Here are some things you should consider doing:

- *WEIGHT LOSS*

  People who undergo natural treatments learn not only how they are cured of their high blood pressure, but also managed to shed extra pounds. When you know the right kind of food to eat, you will minimize your cravings and therefore can lose 1-2 pounds in a week.

- *IMPROVED STAMINA AND ENERGY*

  Because of proper nutrition, you will experience improved stamina and energy and therefore can do things that you can enjoy. When one has a healthy body, life can be better compared to those who don't have a healthy and fit body.

- *REVIVING YOUTHFULNESS*

When you have high blood pressure, you are missing out on significant vitamins and minerals that are needed by the body. Vitamins and minerals like calcium, magnesium, and zinc play a vital role in normalizing your blood pressure. When you have adequate of these substances, then you will feel much younger and alive.

* *CONTROLLING HYPERTENSION*

There are over a thousand listed benefits for exercising and controlling your blood pressure is one of them. Learn a simple exercise, which you can do every day for 20-30 minutes, and you will eventually experience that your blood pressure is going back to normal.

- *No Side Effects!!!*

   Unlike medicine drugs, the only side effect you can get from taking natural remedy is feeling bad about not trying it sooner.

NATURAL WAYS TO CONTROL HIGH BLOOD PRESSURE WITHOUT MEDICATION

Changing lifestyle is said to show a normalized blood pressure in around 86 percent of those who have this disease. Therefore, if you want to reverse your hypertension, you need to normalize your weight. Once you begin to have healthier eating habits, then you can start adapting to the following strategies to beat your hypertension.

- *STEP #1 – WALK, WALK, WALK!*

  Start to walk as much as you can. Work up to walk slowly for longer and longer distances. Try power walking – brisk walking for about 30 minutes a day. This activity can increase your oxygen supply in the body to keep your heart function smoothly and efficiently. As you get used to power walking, try to increase your speed and distance while you increase strength and stamina.

- *STEP #2 – INHALE, EXHALE!*

  Take time to breathe deeply. Sit in a chair with your back straight. Breathe as deeply as you can for five or ten minutes. Stress hormones elevate a kidney enzyme called renin, which raises blood pressure. By slowly deep breathing and expanding your belly, you exhale all the tension out of your body. Adding qigong, tai chi, meditation or yoga to that deep breath is another excellent stress buster.

- *STEP #3 – TAKE MORE POTASSIUM, REDUCE SODIUM IN YOUR DIET*

Watch out for the amount of animal protein in your diet because overeating some of it causes a rise in your body acid levels and diminishes your potassium level. Therefore, it is better to add more naturally potassium-rich foods to your meals such as fresh fruits and vegetables, whole grain, dairy and poultry products, meat, and fish.

High potassium-rich foods include broccoli, halibut, tuna, spinach, parsley, oranges, bananas, avocados, strawberries, crimini mushrooms, Brussels sprouts, kidney beans, tuna, eggplant, apricots, dried prunes, raisins, cantaloupe, honeydew melon, potatoes, peas, squash, chard, sweet potatoes, bell peppers, cucumbers, tomatoes, and cabbage.

Buy as little processed food and limit your sodium intake by buying food that contains a higher level of sodium. You can avoid this by reading food labels, as you will become more aware of the amount of salt in every pack of food that you buy in the grocery store or supermarket. People with high blood pressure are sometimes salt-sensitive. Because there is no available test to show if you are sensitive to salt or not, it is, therefore, essential to be aware of how much salt you are taking so to be able to reduce as much as possible.

- *STEP #4 – ADD COCOA TO YOUR DIET*

A half an ounce of dark chocolate added to your diet contains at least 70 percent cocoa. Dark chocolate contains a substance called "flavanols", which make blood vessel more elastic. The elasticity of blood vessels helps to lower down high blood pressure.

Cocoa flavanols are bioactive derived from cacao beans. Studies on cacao beans disclosed that flavanols could improve cardiovascular functions while lowering the burden on the heart that comes along with aging and heart's stiffening. The study further reveals that the intake of cocoa flavanols reduces the risk of developing cardiovascular diseases.

- *STEP #5 – ALCOHOLIC BEVERAGE HELPS, TOO!*

Having about ¼ -1/2 drink of alcoholic beverage helps to lower your blood pressure. Studies revealed that a small amount of alcoholic drink in a day decreases the risk of heart disease and protects the heart. However, more than that is sure to be detrimental.

- *STEP #6 – AVOID CAFFEINE*

Studies about caffeine show that it causes high blood pressure by tightening blood vessels. This highlights the effects of stress and raises high blood pressure as well. Therefore, you can avoid a blood pressure spikes when you are stressed by using decaf coffee and other drinks.

Drinking hibiscus coffee is associated with a significant decrease in hypertension. A study has proven that drinking 3 cups of hibiscus coffee a day for six weeks brings a substantial change in the level of blood pressure of participants. The Journal of Nutrition had published that hibiscus tea can cause the blood pressure to lower down naturally and was effective in adults who are classified as either mildly hypertensive or pre-hypertensive.

- *STEP #7 – AVOID WORKING TOO MUCH!*

Working for more than 41 hours in a week can add hypertension to the list of health risks since people who works too much tend to eat less healthy food and do not have enough time to exercise. Overload of responsibilities and tasks adds stress to your daily routine, which could later bring you more health issues. Therefore, try to rest as often as you can.

More Alternative Treatments to Include in Your Diet!

There are many other ways to normalize your high blood pressure, and you can include these in your diet. Here are some of them.

- *SELENIUM*

    Selenium, copper, and zinc are just some of the compound elements that can be helpful. Many studies show how people with heart diseases are often deficient of these items. You can have supplements some of these features by taking multi-vitamins in your diet. Sources of selenium are meat, walnuts, Brazil nuts, dark greens, and wheat. Zinc is usually found in beans, meat, and dairy while copper is present in seafood, legumes, nuts, and dark, leafy vegetables.

- *BETA-GLUCAN*

  This substance lowers cholesterol level and likewise reduces blood pressure resulting from high cholesterol. You can get beta-glucan from oat bran and maitake mushroom. This element further aids in moving waste materials out of the human body. A 200-milligram of oat bran (about a teaspoon) to be taken daily can lower hypertension.

- *L'ARGINE*

  By taking 2 grams of L'argine a day can reduce systolic pressure by 20 points after you have taken the supplement for two days. It is primariy due to the amino acid that helps the body to produce nitric acid, which regulates blood pressure and cholesterol.

- *FISH OIL OR FLAXSEED*

Known as Omega 3 fatty acid, fish oil is beneficial for those who are suffering from hypertension. Fish oil protects the heart as well as lowers the blood pressure. For vegetarians, you can try flaxseed. Consuming just a tablespoon of the flaxseed daily can help you lower down your hypertension by nine points.

CHAPTER 6: HERB REMEDIES: HOW CAN THEY HELP TO NORMALIZE YOUR BLOOD PRESSURE

One of the naturally accepted treatments for high blood pressure is the use of herbal as home remedies. The recent increase in the movement away from drug medication is mainly because of the fact that people are fed up with the side effects resulting from the use of drug medication, not to say the costly prescriptions.

HERBAL REMEDIES FOR HIGH BLOOD PRESSURE

- *ARJUNA (TERMINALIA ARJUNA)*

The Arjuna plant is associated with high blood pressure treatment. Its bark is known for its remarkable remedy of the sickness by protecting the heart and stopping the bleeding as well as toughening the muscles in the organ while improving the blood circulation.

Triterpene Glycosides and *Coenzymes Q10* compound substances that help the heart and the arterial blood vessels to function properly are said to be abundant in Arjuna plant. Regular use of this herbal medicine will help eliminate the risk of hypertension and prevent further damage to the heart and the rest of vital organs that are affected by high blood pressure.

- *DANDELION (TARAXACUM OFFICINALE)*

  If you have an issue on fluid retention, dandelion can be useful as it helps increase the urine flow and helps lower blood pressure. One can benefit from the use of dandelions through the elimination of potassium loss, which pharmaceutical diuretics often have. However, make sure that when you use these dandelion leaves, they are not treated with pesticides.

- *CAYENNE (CAPSICUM ANNUM)*

  Cayenne aids in thinning of the blood, thus lowering your blood pressure. Just use the hot Mexican or Thai seeds like those used in Serrano or African Bird Peppers, which are among the hottest of the cayenne products.

  To use cayenne for remedy, just take a cup of lukewarm water mixed with one teaspoon of cayenne pepper. Drink the solution for maintenance.

- *GINGER (ZINGIBER OFFICINALE)*

Another herb that is commonly used as a cooking spice is ginger. Though we often consume this home kitchen ingredient, yet most are not aware of its health benefits, including regulating high blood pressure. Ginger is very useful in improving blood flow, treating nausea, relaxing muscles of the arteries, facilitating easy digestion, and easing morning sickness.

Garlic may come in various forms including dry roots, capsules, fresh roots, oils, liquid extracts, powders, supplements, etc. You can eat garlic raw or add it to your delectable dishes.

While ginger is proclaimed as safe and effective for hypertension, some people may experience some possible side effects which you must be cautious of – Allergic reactions, gastric disturbance, heartburn problems or mouth irritation.

* *GUGGUL (COMMIPHORA WIGHTII)*

Primarily, this herb grows in India but can also be found in other countries in Central Asia and Northern Africa. Studies indicate that this amazing herb can reduce bad cholesterol LDL and likewise address health issues related to psoriasis, arteriosclerotic vascular disease, and cardiac ischemia.

* *GARLIC (ALLIUM SATIVUM)*

For a long time, we have recognized garlic as an aromatic ingredient we used for food seasoning. However, we failed to realize that garlic lowers down our blood pressure by ten percent. Even when it's in the form of gel capsules, garlic still has the same effect.

Garlic also possesses the capability to lessen blood clotting and clears your arteries of bad cholesterols and plaques. For better performance, daily consumption of 1 or 2 cloves for 90 days is enough to prevent and minimize the effects of high blood pressure. It can either be eaten raw or included in your meals.

- *REISHI (GANODERMA LUCID)*

  This is one species of mushroom associated with lowering of blood pressure. The mushroom is almost inedible but available in capsule form.

- *HAWTHORN (CRATAEGUS APP)*

  Hawthorn causes arterial walls to relax and dilate, and it can take many weeks or months to show any effect.

- *HAWTHORN (CRATAEGUS LAEVIGATA)*

  Hawthorn is beneficial in widening arterial blood vessels, preventing the growth of atherosclerosis, decreasing cholesterol levels, enhancing blood circulation, and regulating heartbeat.

  You can consume this herb by drinking it in tea form using its dried leaves and flowers. You may also include hawthorn berry supplements in your dietary plan. Whatever way you use, you can experience a 2.60 HG reduction in your blood pressure level. All these results established hawthorn as a highly trusted herbal treatment for blood pressure.

- *CELERY (APIUM GRAVEOLENS)*

Celery has been used as a remedy since the early age, and it occupies a unique herbal treatment for blood pressure. It aids in increasing the flow of urine. Indians have used it in their daily life having recognized celery as one of the best remedies for high blood pressure.

- *COCOA (THEOBROMA CACAO)*

Another fantastic herb that is associated with lowering high blood pressure efficiently is the Cocoa. It works as antioxidants like tea and red wine. According to researchers, a daily dose of 3.5

ounces of cocoa is effective as taking a daily dose of high blood pressure medication.

- *VALERIAN (VALERIANA OFFICINALIS)*

  Valerian relaxes the smooth muscles lining the arterial walls by preventing them from constricting.

- *BROCCOLI (BRASSICA OLERACEA VAR. ITALICA) AND DARK LEAFY GREENS*

  Broccoli and dark leafy vegetables are high in vitamins and minerals that are an essential need for people with high blood pressure. Magnesium and calcium are found in abundance in broccoli and other dark leafy vegetables.

- *TURMERIC (LUCUMA LONGA)*

Turmeric, the spice, is often used in curries. It has anti-inflammatory and antioxidant properties that lower cholesterol level and strengthen body vessels as well as reduce blood pressure.

- *GINGKO BILOBA*

  Gingko Biloba is known Chinese herbal remedy for hypertension that improves circulation of the blood and dilates arteries. It also enhances memory and makes one mentally alert.

- *OLIVE LEAF EXTRACT*

  The extract derived from the olive leaf is used as a remedy for high blood pressure to combat irregular heartbeat or what is called "arrhythmia."

- *JAUNDICE BERRY*

  With this herbal remedy, blood flow is facilitated to run smoothly in the arteries by dilating blood vessels through the release of tension on the arteries.

- *CAYENNE*

  Cayenne is known as the best herb for high blood pressure next to garlic. To get the best results, choose the hottest of the cayenne spices. Cayenne is known to result in proper control of blood pressure.

- *RED CLOVER*

  People with high blood pressure tend to have their blood thickened resulting to the extra effort of the heart in pumping blood through the vessels. The pressure therefore against the arteries is heightened causing hypertension. Red clover is best for thinning blood hence, lowering blood pressure, and improving blood circulation. To be efficiently used, the red clover needs to be in good state – blossoms must remain purple. Brown coloured clover is dry and has lost their effectiveness.

- *ALFALFA*

  Alfalfa helps in softening hardened arteries while reducing high blood pressure. It plays a vital role in hypertension treatment.

- *PARSLEY*

  Parsley is best in maintaining blood circulation and the whole circulatory system of the body while it lowers high blood pressure.

- *GOOSEBERRY*

  Known as "Amla" in India, gooseberry can be consumed with honey in its juice form. Take 1-2 tablespoon daily on an empty stomach as is a primarily beneficial to people with high blood pressure.

- *ONION AND HONEY*

A mixture of onion juice and honey can do wonders for people with high blood pressure. Drinking two teaspoons a day of this mixture can reverse the effect of high blood pressure and helps you return to a stable blood pressure.

- *FENUGREEK SEED (TRIGONELLA FOENUM-GRAECUM)*

  Seeds from this plant are known to carry various health benefits including the following:

- LOWERS BLOOD CHOLESTEROL

  Studies have proven that fenugreek helps in reducing cholesterol level, particularly that of LDL or low-density lipoprotein. The herb is known to be enriched with steroidal saponins, which is associated with the absorption of cholesterol and triglycerides.

- REDUCES RISKS OF HEART DISEASE

  Fenugreek leaves contain a high amount of potassium that counters the adverse effects of sodium in the body to help control heartbeat rate and blood pressure.

- ## KEEPS YOU IN SHAPE

  When you include fenugreek in your diet by chewing soaked seeds in the morning on an empty stomach, the natural fiber in the fenugreek can fill up and causes your stomach to swell, suppressing your appetite. This aids you in attaining your weight loss goals, as you also tend to lose your cravings for foods.

All the above conditions are beneficial and will help you naturally lower your high blood pressure.

Chapter 7: Stress Management: Empowering Mind and Body

It's still debatable whether long-term blood pressure and stress are connected. However, taking measures to manage and reduce your stress dramatically benefits your overall health including your blood pressure.

The Connection Between Stress and Long-term High Blood Pressure

While experts cannot define the direct relationship between these two, it's proven that stressful events can cause temporary increase in blood pressure. What you can do to avoid long-term high blood pressure is to take preventive measures that will benefit your health in both mind and body.

Exercising is a drug-free way of helping you lower your blood pressure. It reduces your stress levels as it releases endorphins, which are essential in making you feel good about yourself and the things around you. For instance, you can exercise 3-5 times a week for about half an hour to reduce your stress level. Other physical activities such as doing household chores, gardening, dancing, swimming, or jogging can also increase your breathing and heart rates, generating benefits in rendering your blood pressure under control.

Remember that under stressful situations, your body produces a rush of hormones, which can cause your heart to beat faster for a while and narrowing your blood vessels in the process. As we mentioned earlier, there's no absolute proof that stress directly results in long-term blood pressure but behaviours such as overeating, smoking, substance abuse and observing poor sleeping habits can all contribute to high blood pressure. Overtime, these series of temporary sharp increases in blood pressure can put you in danger of having a long-term high blood pressure.

On the other hand, stress-related health conditions such as isolation, anxiety, and depression, which can be connected to heart disease may not be related to high blood pressure at all. The reason may be because of the hormones that are produced during the stressful moments.

These hormones can then damage the arteries, exposing you to the risks of heart disease. Additionally, if you are stressed or depressed, you also tend to neglect yourself. This includes the probability of not taking necessary medications that can control your high blood pressure and heart condition.

ACTIVITIES THAT CAN REDUCE BLOOD PRESSURE

Stress management is a skill that can help you in a lot of ways. Mastering it can help you live a healthy lifestyle that can benefit your overall health—both mind and boy—including the regulation of your blood pressure. The following steps may help you get started in how to handle your stress:

MAKE YOUR SCHEDULE SIMPLE

One of the most challenging things most of us experience is how to simplify our schedule. Usually, we tend to procrastinate only to find ourselves in a rush to finish our work, projects, assignments, etc. With this hustle and bustle, it's quite reasonable that our body accepts this as stress, which isn't good for our body when accumulated over time.

Eliminate or curtail additional activities that take up a lot of your time. For example, chatting with your friends on Facebook takes a great deal of your morning schedule. Instead of doing this, you can choose a more time-worthy activity wherein you can move around your body or exercise your mind, such as trying to meditate.

BE CONSCIOUS OF YOUR BREATHING

Breathing is essential for us; after all, we breathe to live. When we breathe, each cell in our body takes in the supply of oxygen that contributes to the production of energy in our system. It also allows us to get rid of the toxins that our body must eliminate to stay healthy.

Unfortunately, most of us take breathing for granted. Busy schedule and fast-paced lifestyle contribute more to our neglect in taking deep breaths which are very important in our health.

You can do simple breathing exercises by doing deep inhalation and exhalation all throughout the day. Take a few deep breaths and let your body relax, letting go of the stressors accumulating in your body. This process allows you to intake oxygen and feeds the cells of your body the much-needed supply necessary for your survival.

Do Regular Work Out

In this modern age wherein computers and various gadgets dominate our lifestyle, we tend to be sedentary. Remember that physical activity is a natural stress reliever. With the advice of your doctor, you can plan your exercises starting from simple activities such as walking or jogging. You can also try these various activities:

- Doing household chores and gardening
- Climbing the stairs
- Walking (in the park or any relaxing place)
- Dancing
- Playing tennis, basketball, or dodgeball

MEDITATE

Meditation has been proven to benefit the health of both our mind and body. It helps us to relax and have that inner calm that is essential to achieving balance.

Back in 2008, Massachusetts General Hospital doctor Randy Zusman asked his patients with high blood pressure to undertake a three-month-long meditation-base relaxation program. These patients regularly took medication to control their high blood pressure. After three months, 40 out of 60 patients displayed a remarkable drop in their blood pressure levels.

As a result, they were able to lessen their medication intake. The scientific explanation about this is that as the body and mind enter the state of relaxation, nitric oxide can then be formed resulting in the opening of blood vessels, regulating the flow of blood pressure.

Yoga helps you to control your blood pressure. In doing regular stretches, your muscles can become flexible resulting in controlled blood pressure without the use of medications. Stretching exercises develop a series of physiological reactions that may inhibit the stiffening of arteries due to aging.

DEVELOP GOOD SLEEPING HABITS

When you are deprived of sleep, you usually gain weight due to the lowering of your *leptin* (the hormone in charge of prompting your brain that you already had enough food eaten) hormone levels and an increase of the biochemical called *ghrelin* which intensifies your appetite to eat.

This bodily reaction dramatically affects your eating behavior, making you intake high amounts of calories which your body doesn't need.

Additionally, sleep deprivation also makes your body release higher levels of insulin after you eat, boosting fat storage and exposing you to a higher risk of having type-2 diabetes.

Sleep plays a vital role in repairing and healing your blood vessels as well as your heart. Lack of it promotes high blood pressure, stroke and heart disease.

According to one study of Harvard Medical School, patients with high blood pressure may experience the hike of their blood pressure levels all throughout the next day upon staying late the night before. To help yourself fight off sleep deprivation, here are the best steps that you should observe:

- Consume caffeine only in mornings.

- Set aside your mobile devices and other gadgets after dinner.

- Observe a consistent wake-up schedule.

- Avoid using sedatives like Valium, Nyquil, Ambien or even alcohol.

- Take a 15-minute nap every afternoon instead of drinking coffee.

BE OPTIMISTIC

Having a positive mindset and attitude dramatically helps in promoting your overall health. When you're mind is relaxed, your body automatically creates balance and harmony leading to good health—and regulating your blood pressure levels is one of the benefits of having this inner calm. Quite some studies also show that being optimistic tend to give a person a quality and long life. For instance, a happy and contented person who enjoys laughing in the company of his loved ones manages to lead a long life compared to those who suffer depression or have a negative outlook on life.

According to some studies, there is an association between the positive outlook and lower blood pressure. Individuals who have a positive mindset tend to have controlled blood pressure levels; whereas, those who look towards life in a negative perspective have the highest risk of developing high blood pressure. Moreover, positive individuals have the lower percentage of exposing themselves into evolving into cardiovascular disease.

Therefore, if you want to enjoy a quality life until your old age, it's time to recreate your mindset. You can always start with little things. In other words, you can marvel at the little things nature gives us like the sunlight, warmth, the sky or even the moon during the night.

Be conscious of your inner voice and how you talk to yourself. Avoid talking about your mistakes or highlighting your worries. Before you are tempted to do that, give yourself some space and assess the situation. While you can see unfavourable aspects, you always have the choice to shed on that matter. Don't forget to laugh in every chance you have. A good one can help lessen your mental burden, even making it easier for you to handle challenging problems.

CHAPTER 8: HOW MEDITATION CAN HELP IN LOWERING HIGH BLOOD PRESSURE

In addition to the conventional methods of combating high blood pressure, Mindfulness-Based Reduction Technique (MBRS) is gaining followers and practitioners all over the world. By incorporating mindfulness meditation into your lifestyle along with physical fitness activity and weight management, your goal of reducing high blood pressure is achieved and thereby reverse its effect on your body.

According to a research study, to curb blood pressure and ward off hypertension, it is critical to keep your mind away from stress and anxiety.

Researchers from Case Western University School of Medicine conducted a study on hundred of patients with hypertension aging 30-60 years old. The program consisted of 8 sessions covering 2 ½ hours each. Participants were then asked to meditate using the body scan exercise for 45 minutes in six days per week. The study resulted in a significant outcome with the result indicating a 1.9-mm Hg decrease in diastolic blood pressure (DBP) and 4.8-mm Hg decrease in systolic blood pressure (SBP). The findings were published in the Psychosomatic Medicine Journal.

In a recent study on blood pressure, distress and coping, it was revealed that through a selected mind-body intervention, a decrease in blood pressure was detected relative to increased coping and decreased psychological distress in young adults conducive to high blood pressure.

Based on these studies, it was proven that meditation could be useful in lowering the level of blood pressure while combating the ill effects of stress and anxiety in the human body.

As you resolve to shift to a healthier lifestyle choice, you must incorporate meditation into your everyday routine. Making a habit of practicing daily or doing meditation exercises even for just 20 minutes is sure to make a big difference on how your body moves, how your mind thinks, and how your body feels.

When your mind and emotions are calm and controllable, you're in a better position to face all the challenges in your life and the goals that you have set for yourself – which in this case happens to be regulating your blood pressure to a reasonable level.

Those negative feelings including worry, anxiety, and fear plus the regular occurrence of stress as you are regularly exposed to various stressors can be significantly relieved by a daily practice of meditation. As your mind is cleared of muddled thoughts, keeping you stuck in unhealthy behaviors, you will be surprised to see how you would see life in a different viewpoint. All the changes in your life always begin in your mind.

Your mind always has the power over your body – from the tip of your hair down to the tip of your toes.

Being able to control your mind and tame it so you can lead it to where you want is an efficient way of calming your overall sense so as not to send your heart beating or pumping as it usually does. When you can do this, then you are getting rid of the stressors that tend to send your blood pressure up.

Rather than doing the same routine using the same mindset and results that are disappointing, meditation allows you to set the stages for some significant shift in your life, and this includes, primarily your health.

MANAGING YOUR HEALTH, SAVING YOUR LIFE!

Just as human illness is relatively stress-related, meditation works well to relieve you from stress. It likewise helps in treating illnesses. Not only mediation resolve the issue on high blood pressure or hypertension risks, but it is also associated with the relief of the following diseases:

- Skin disorders

- Mild depression

- Pre-menstrual syndrome and dysmenorrhea

- Sleeping apnea and fatigue

- Recurring pain including headaches

- Respiratory issues like asthma and emphysema

- Rheumatoid Arthritis (RA) symptoms

- Gastrointestinal distress

- Irritable bowel syndrome

Health and medical condition like the ones we have here will undoubtedly deprive you of the vitality and live a life of fun and enjoyment. When you let stress weight you down as you are burdened with anxiety and negative thoughts and emotions, it stresses that is in control and not you!

Could there be more satisfying than having a cure for a stress-related illness that is natural? This is what meditation is offering you – A life of happiness – free from the claw of this deadly sickness.

A WAY TO DO YOUR MEDITATION EXERCISE

To start, find a comfortable place to do your exercise. Though old-timers can do it anywhere and would find it easy to achieve their meditation goal anywhere and anytime, beginners can get easily distracted; hence, you need a more quiet and serene place to meditate. You can either sit on a chair or the floor as long as you feel comfortable and relaxed. If you need something to soothe your senses, prepare some music.

Start by closing your eyes or just focus your attention on something like maybe the floor near where you are sitting. Then start breathing in and out gently, trying to feel the air as it passes through your nostrils and runs through every part of your body before you slowly take it out through your mouth, Feel every moment – either you focus on your breathing, or you focus on the object of your attention.

If you are closing your eyes, imagine of something – an image, an object, a mantra or anything you want to connect with. If you find your mind wandering out of focus, slowly get it back to being focused without judging yourself. The goal here is to be able to control your thinking to focus on something and not get affected emotionally but just silently look at it at the present moment.

Focusing on your breathing gives you a new awareness of your life, and while you are doing this activity, you may be able to grasp a new meaning to your existence. This could be a simple and quite exercise that could last for a few minutes, but out of it, something new – an insight maybe will be revealed to you in a spur of a moment.

Short as it is, you could not imagine the benefits this meditation exercise can bring you – physically, mentally, emotionally, and spiritually. It is for this reason that more and more people resort back to transcendental or mindfulness meditation as a way of treating stress to reverse the effects of high blood pressure or minimize the risks of more severe health problems.

Ideally, set aside 15-30 minutes a day for meditation so calm down your senses and prepare them for facing the daily struggles and challenges in life. This way, your body won't feel threatened and set itself to a fight or flight mode which causes it to produce some hormonal change in your body, sending your heart to build more pressure and forcing the arterial wall to break.

There are some online resources and tools like the Insight CD System, which you can set up by yourself and so a quick meditation session for 20 minutes or more depending on your preference.

While listening to the CD, you can teach your brain to work n synchronization –that is, training your left and right side of the brain to work in consonance to create a comprehensive distribution of electrical activity and energy patterns throughout your mind instead of having it confined to limited areas. This tool is designed in agreement with the result of a study which indicates that this full brain synchronization is active at times of intense creativity, clarity, and inspiration.

To sum this up, whether you are doing meditation without the use of the Insight audio CD or any tool like this, make sure that that you incorporate the meditation exercise in your daily activities. Make this a habit, not only to regulate your high blood pressure but a part of a healthy lifestyle. It's a simple step, but its lasting result can have a profound and lasting effect on your overall physical health and mental wellbeing.

CONCLUSION

A significant number of hypertension sufferers are now getting tired of experiencing the debilitating effects of drug prescriptions and medication that most opted to resort back to the natural remedies. Now that many are asking if the natural way of treating high blood pressure works, proven studies answer this question with a big "YES!"

However, natural treatment is a holistic approach that needs to be consolidated into your lifestyle to be able to benefit from it entirely. It does not answer to only one area of your life but needs to make a thorough overhauling of your wellbeing.

Now that you have become aware of the extent that natural remedies can do to your goal of bringing down to the reasonable level your high blood pressure, you can use this knowledge to regulate your blood pressure and manage your hypertension to prevent the onset of other complications or more severe illnesses.

High blood pressure can be a silent killer only if you neglect to give enough attention to your lifestyle. It's not high blood that kills, but it's your failure to create a healthy lifestyle that can give you a better, safer, and longer life!

The next step is for you to **join our email newsletter** to receive updates on any upcoming new book releases or promotions. You can sign-up for free and as a bonus, you will also receive our "*7 Fitness Mistakes You Don't Know You're Making*" book! This bonus book breaks down many of the most common fitness mistakes and will demystify many of the complexities and science of getting into shape. Having all this fitness knowledge and science organized into an actionable step-by-step book will help you get started in the right direction in your fitness journey! To join our free email newsletter and grab your free book, please visit the link and signup: **www.hmwpublishing.com/gift**

Finally, if you enjoyed this book, then I would like to ask you for a favor, would you be kind enough to leave a review for this book? It would be greatly appreciated!

Thank you and good luck in your journey!

Type 2 Diabetes Cookbook & Action Plan

The Ultimate Beginner's Diabetic Diet Cookbook & Action Plan Guide to Reverse Pre-diabetes - Quick & Easy Delicious Healthy Type 2 Diabetic Recipes

By *Jennifer Louissa*

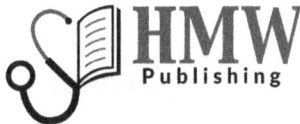

HMW Publishing

For more great books visit:

HMWPublishing.com

Table of Contents

Introduction

Truth be told -- diabetes is tantamount to stories of struggles. And the very first struggle was to process the fact that you are in the pre-diabetic stage. It's never easy. The more you think about the disease, the more you get inundated with 'what if's'.

One reality that people living with diabetes need to deal with is how to come to terms with the disease on a daily basis. What to do? What not to do? What to eat? How not to suffer? And the list of questions continues. It can get pretty tiring at some point, especially when you are completely lost in the process.

But, one thing is certain -- you need to cultivate determination throughout the process. Yes, you need to stick your neck out and deal with it. You need to overcome your fear of this disease to be able to manage it.

Most importantly, you need an Action Plan.

In other words, you need that weapon to destruct what could destruct you from the inside. Yes, an Action plan that entails your micro goals. Your ultimate goal is to reverse your pre-diabetes stage. Your micro goals, on the other hand, should direct your steps on how to strike a balance among your food, physical activities, and medication to combat the repercussions of this condition.

Bear in mind that diabetes is a lifelong disease. When you are unable to reverse the pre-diabetic stage, you will find yourself battling with a bigger monster. Love yourself more, and this book will help and guide you on how you can do this correctly. With the right action plan in hand, you will be able to take charge of your life.

Also, before you get started, I recommend you **joining our email newsletter** to receive updates on any upcoming new book releases or promotions. You can sign-up for free, and as a bonus, you will receive a free gift. Our "*Health & Fitness Mistakes You Don't Know You're Making*" book! This book has been written to demystify, expose the top do's and don'ts and to finally equip you with the information you need to get in the best shape of your life. Due to the overwhelming amount of mis-information and lies told by magazines and self-proclaimed "gurus", it's becoming harder and harder to get reliable information to get in shape. As opposed to having to go through dozens of biased, unreliable and un-trustworthy sources to get your health & fitness information. Everything you need to help you has been broken down in this book for you to easily follow and to immediately get results to achieve your desired fitness goals in the shortest amount of time. Once again, to join our free email newsletter and to receive a free copy of this valuable book, please visit the link and signup now: **www.hmwpublishing.com/gift**

Chapter 1: The truth about diabetes

What Diabetes Is and What It Is Not?

What is diabetes - this is probably the very first question that crossed your mind when your doctor told you that you are in the 'pre-diabetic' stage. You have probably heard about the disease several times, but do not know what it is or how it develops.

When we eat, the food is processed and turns into glucose (sugar). Our body then uses the glucose as a source of energy. Our pancreas, on the other hand, produces insulin which enables the glucose to get into the cells of the body.

When you are diagnosed with diabetes or at the pre-diabetic stage, it could mean one of these two: either your body does not produce sufficient insulin or that your body is unable to use insulin well. When this happens, the glucose then builds up in your blood, and this when you develop diabetes.

Diabetes, by simple definition, means that your sugar level in the blood gets too high. Although your blood needs to have sugar in it to energize you, too much of it can be detrimental to your overall health. Specifically, it can damage several organs in your body including the kidneys, heart, eyes, and the nerves. The word itself pertains to the chronic disease that involves sugar levels and sweets which is why the next word you often see with *diabetes* is *mellitus.*

The word *Mellitus,* on the other hand, literally means sweet, sweetened, or honey – something along the line of sugary sweetness. The disease is officially called *Diabetes Mellitus,* but often, the medical world can do without including *mellitus* because everyone already knows what the word diabetes means and its general nature as a disease. So, to clarify any possible confusion in the future, *diabetes* and *diabetes mellitus* are the same.

Are You at Risk? Check this List!

Before we discuss the risk factors, let's have a quick glimpse at the two types of diabetes to understand better who are more prone to this disease.

Overall, there are two types of Diabetes, namely: Type 1 and Type 2. Another type is referred to as Gestational Diabetes which develops during pregnancy. About 1 out of 10 people inflicted with diabetes has Type 1 and is more common in children or younger adults. People with Type 1 diabetes tend to become dependent on injectable insulin as their pancreas can produce very little to no insulin at all.

The main reason behind this phenomenon is still unknown, and several types of research are on-going. This is to learn what prompts the body to attack the pancreas' beta cells and stop producing insulin. About 90% of people with diabetes suffer Type 2. In these cases, the pancreas produces insulin, but the body is not able to utilize the hormone very well. People with this condition discover about the case usually after the age of 30.

People who are likely to develop diabetes are those with the following conditions:

- A family history of diabetes
- Has a history of gestational diabetes
- Overweight or obese

Let's take a closer look at the different risk factors and what each of them means for the different types of diabetes. Take note of these and use the list for self-assessment.

Risk Factors for Type 1 Diabetes Mellitus

While the principal cause of this disorder has not been identified yet, the factors that increase one's chance of developing it have been defined. These include the following:

History of the Family

This means that you have a higher chance of developing it if at least of your parents or siblings has it.

Dietary Factor and Eating Habits

Your choice of food plays a crucial role in the possible development of diabetes. Moreover, other related risk factors include minimal consumption of Vitamin D, early intake of cow's milk formula, and also the consumption of cereals before becoming four months old.

Environmental Factors

A person's exposure to specific viral illnesses may also trigger the development of this metabolic disease. The presence of auto-antibodies in your system. This is also referred to as a self-damaging immune system.

Geographic Factors

It has been found that people from some countries are more at risk of developing Type 1 Diabetes. These include Sweden and Finland.

Risk Factors for Type 2 Diabetes Mellitus

Weight

Simply put, the more or thicker fatty tissues you have in your body, the more resistant you become to insulin.

Family History

As with Type 1, you are likely to develop diabetes if at least one of the immediate family members has diabetes.

Sedentary Lifestyle

In order words, being inactive -- physically inactive, for that matter, makes you even more prone to diabetes. This is because physical activity prompts your body to make use of glucose as your source of energy.

Age

Basically, the older you get, the more exposed you are to the risks of developing such disease. Reasons for this may include the change in your lifestyle as you tend to exercise less and consequently gain weight.

Race

One of the biggest mysteries behind diabetes is that individual races are more prone to it. These include Asian-Americans, Hispanics, American Africans, and Hispanics.

High Blood Pressure or Hypertension

Having a blood pressure that is over 140/80 millimeters of mercury is also associated with the risks of developing Diabetes as well.

Polycystic Ovarian Syndrome

This is a common condition that women with irregular menstruation, obesity, and excessive hair growth have. Those who are inflicted with this condition are also exposed to higher risks of developing diabetes.

Abnormal levels of triglyceride and cholesterol levels

If you high levels of 'bad' cholesterol and triglyceride, you are at risks of developing diabetes. This also means that your 'good' cholesterol or HDL is at a low level.

Gestational Diabetes

Women who had gestational diabetes while pregnant are also at risk of developing Type 2 later in life. Also, if you gave birth to relatively heavier babies (i.e., About 4 kilograms or above), you are also at risk.

Highlighting Facts and Dispelling Myths

1. Keeping diabetes in check is as easy as 1, 2, 3

First things first, diabetes is not to be taken lightly. Just like cardiovascular disease that comes to you like a silent killer and then hits you without warning, diabetes is known for creeping up on you as well. And don't ever think that the worst is over after being diagnosed with diabetes. The worst is just about to start because being aware of it doesn't stop it from attacking you surprisingly again. So, no, it is never easy to keep diabetes in check.

2. Having diabetes means you'll have to have insulin shots

Well, that depends. If you are diagnosed with diabetes type 1 then, sadly, there is no other choice for you but to have insulin shots because it is ALWAYS required. Now, if you have diabetes type 2, insulin shots are not needed every time. If your diabetes is controllable with some other medicines mainly to be taken orally, then there is no need for you to inject insulin. But, if not, then you will have to go for the injection method.

3. Sugar is the main culprit

While sugar is often INVOLVED when a person is diagnosed with diabetes, it does not mean that it is always the cause. Sometimes, it is just a contributing factor. The truth is, our bodies also require sugar. It does not only help us store energy, which is the function that gets messed up when a person has diabetes, but it is a vital part of our DNA or *deoxyribonucleic acid* – the primary material that carries all of our genetic information.

Also, diets that involve sugar also depend on the weight of the person consuming it. So if your diet is quite high in sugar, but you can maintain your average weight and insulin levels, you will not get diabetes because what many people think is "high" is actually what your body requires. However, if your weight is a little on the heavier side with a family history of diabetes, which is also a significant factor in being diagnosed with the disease, and your blood sugar is beyond reasonable then you should be a little careful with your sugar intake.

So, rejoice, people of the world! You can still enjoy sugar and sweets. Just make sure that you do not snack on it. To be sure, always see to it that you **include** them in your meals in proper servings or portioning.

4. Being overweight makes you an automatic diabetes type 2 patient

Not exactly. Let me sort it out for you. Being overweight is a *serious risk* factor for developing diabetes type 2, yes. However it is just a *risk factor,* and it does not guarantee that you are, indeed, suffering from diabetes.

5. Obese or fat people are the only ones who get diabetes

This is so untrue. It is possible for thin people to develop diabetes as well if they are unable to control the levels of their blood sugar. Things only become worse especially if they have a family history of diabetes and it starts manifesting because of their ages, too. So, no. Just because you are fat does not mean you have diabetes and just because you are thin does not mean you are safe from having diabetes. Diabetes is way beyond *just the weight*.

6. Diabetes is incurable

That is what some doctors back then would say to you but, it is not entirely accurate. Diabetes *is only incurable* if you are not planning to change your lifestyle and diet. However, if you are willing to do anything just so you can live a couple more years to enjoy life with your loved ones, then definitely diabetes is curable. It is only a matter of discipline, priorities, diet, and lifestyle. I understand, it is easier said than done, but you have to start somewhere, right?

7. Diabetes is not serious

Okay, so we have settled the fact that diabetes is curable, but that does not mean it is not severe. **Diabetes is a chronic disease**, and if not appropriately managed or left unattended, it gets worse over time.

Now, before I get to the part where I emphasize the gravity of diabetes as a disease, let me explain the word *chronic* to give you a general feel of urgency when it comes to chronic diseases.

- Chronic – we hear this word from our doctors too often that we have learned just to ignore it and the message that it is trying to convey. For someone who has an inkling about the words *chronic disease,* they would think it merely pertains to a condition that has been ongoing for quite some time. This statement is true, *however,* only partly.

Chronic disease pertains to the kind of illness that has been ongoing for quite some time in a very persistent manner. It causes long-term effects that may include complications that are altogether difficult to get rid of.

That being said, let us now return to the topic at hand – diabetes. Apart from the fact that it is chronic, diabetes in advance cases brings in its wake a myriad of complications such as kidney diseases, cardiovascular diseases *also known as heart diseases*, and other combo diseases that you would not want to worry yourself with anymore.

So, please, if you do not want to make it more complicated than it already is, do not take it lightly and act as soon as you can.

8. People with diabetes do not have insulin in their bodies

This is a baseless theory. Diabetes has two types, each with their characteristics.

Diabetes type 1 –

- Incapable of insulin production due to the immune system *incorrectly attacking* the pancreatic beta cells responsible for insulin production.

- Usually diagnosed while the patient is in his childhood.

- Does not often have something to do with being overweight.

- **Always** require insulin shots to control the disease.

- Often involves normal levels of ketone upon diagnosis.

Before we move on to the other type of diabetes, let us first talk about what *ketones* are.

- Ketones are molecules that are produced by the liver *when* a person is not eating correctly (*high sugar diet, excessive carbohydrate restriction, improper diet leading to starvation*), when doing an exercise that is too strenuous for long periods of time, and when suffering from insulin deficiency or diabetes type 1. Ketones are what comes after your body burns fat to keep you fueled.

What does it have to do with diabetes?

Since a diabetic's body does not produce insulin, which helps convert sugar into energy, glucose or sugar that is not converted enters your bloodstream. So, instead of joining the cells, glucose stays in the bloodstream coating your blood cells in the process and coats the insides of your arteries as well.

The results:

- Your blood becomes sugary sweet **and thick** *(This is why in advance cases of diabetes, you might see some patients being surrounded by ants, literally.)*

- Your arteries become narrower, or worse, clogged

- Thick blood + narrow arteries = high blood pressure **OR**

- Thick blood + clogged arteries = atherosclerosis (arteries becoming hard due to clogging formed by thick blood), **OR** an aneurysm (ruptured arteries due to blood not being able to pass through because of the clog), **OR** stroke.

Such a horrible equation, but it is the truth, and the explanation is far from being done.

Going back to the topic, our cells still needs something to burn so, burn they go. But, in the absence of glucose (*since glucose is busy doing nothing while staying in the bloodstream where they are not supposed to be in*), the next best thing that our cells choose to burn are fats. And so, ketones *or **acids*** are produced.

So, what?

Well, the body goes through **ketoacidosis**. Ketoacidosis is when your body produces too much acid that disturbs the body's natural pH.

What is pH?

pH is the unit of measurement of alkaline and acid in the body. The body's average pH level **should** stay between degrees of 7.30 to 7.45, meaning *slightly* alkalic. Anything below 7.30 level says your body is acidic or is undergoing ketoacidosis. Anything above 7.45 level means your body is too alkalic. .

If a body goes through ketoacidosis and not treated immediately, it will lead to *diabetic coma* because the blood sugar is either too high (*hyperglycemia*) or too low (*hypoglycemia*). This state pushes the body and the blood sugar to extremes and if not immediately attended to, can lead to death.

<u>Diabetes type 2</u> –

✓ Has insulin in the body, it's just that the body has developed resistance to it rendering the insulin useless.

✓ People in middle age are the ones often diagnosed with the disease.

✓ Being overweight plays a significant role in this disease.

✓ involves high levels of cholesterol and blood pressure

✓ in some cases, can be controlled with oral medications

✓ can be treated initially with proper lifestyle

and diet

9. Being diagnosed with diabetes calls for dialysis

Renal disease or failure (*kidney disease or kidney failure*) is a complication of unmonitored diabetes. Meaning, if you take good care of yourself after being diagnosed with diabetes, monitor what needs monitoring and control what needs controlling so that you can avoid having to manage complications on top of diabetes.

10. Insulin takes care of it all

This is not true. Taking insulin, in the case of diabetes type 2, makes sure that you have the right amount of energy converted from sugar and then adequately utilized. It means your diet has to cooperate with your insulin intake to make sure that your body is not stuffing itself full of unused insulin and sugar that eventually gets mixed in your blood making it thicker, leading to advanced diabetes and even heart disease. If you do not change your diet and lifestyle, then don't be surprised if your diabetes gets worse faster than you can imagine.

11. Diabetes type 1 is worse than diabetes type 2

Being diagnosed with any of the two is bad enough. If you do not budge to keep your diabetes in control, whether it is type 1 or 2, it will finish you off like the silent killer it is – fast and without remorse.

12. Insulin causes blindness

Not true. Diabetes, if left unmonitored and uncontrolled, causes blindness. Ignorance is a complication of diabetes in its advanced stage, much like kidney failure and heart disease. If blindness occurred because a person used insulin, it's highly likely that the diabetes of that person has been ignored for quite a long time.

13. Diabetes is a pancreatic disorder

Diabetes is not a pancreatic disorder. It depends on the type of diabetes that you have, but if you have diabetes type 1, then what it is, is an *autoimmune disease.*

First, pancreatic disorder *or pancreatitis* is an inflammation of the pancreas. ***Any medical term that has a suffix of –itis pertains to inflammation.***

In the case of diabetes, the pancreas has long been inflamed and too severe to be even considered merely a pancreatic disorder. Fact is, pancreatic disorder leads to diabetes if left untreated. Think of it like this: ***Acute***

Pancreatic Inflammation (*acute, meaning short-term and abrupt onset of the disease*) is the seed, ***Chronic Pancreatic Inflammation*** is the seedling, and that one humongous monster tree is ***Diabetes***.

How so? Like I mentioned awhile ago, in diabetes type 1, the immune system reacts incorrectly by attacking the pancreas leading to the inability of our body to produce insulin. As for diabetes type 2, it is considered a metabolic disorder, but research is being performed because the medical world is looking at the possibility of *autoimmune disease* angle

Reversing Pre-Diabetes with Nutrition. Is it Possible?

To cut to the chase, yes it is possible. The earlier you learn about your condition, the better it is.

To reverse pre-diabetes, you have to maintain a diet that is tailor-fit to you with the help of your doctor. Below is a general guideline for reversing pre-diabetes.

- **Take it seriously.**

  Pre-diabetes is just a notch away from getting actual diabetes, and if you do not treat it correctly this time, chances are you will also have a problem with *practical* diabetes in the future. Do not wait for it to happen and be as precautious as you can. It might be a little confusing to adjust to this kind of lifestyle, but this is better than getting sick, right?

- **Monitor your blood sugar at least 2-3 times a week.**

  Pre-diabetes patients shouldn't only stick to A1C tests. You should also make sure that you know what is happening to your blood sugar weekly. This is to help you find out if your current diet is helping or not. Customize your diet with your doctor as soon as you can, to smoothly reverse pre-diabetes.

- **Watch what you eat.**

  You can still enjoy a cheat day despite being in this pre-diabetes state, but you have to be vigilant and disciplined for the rest of the week. You see, keeping your body in a healthier shape can help you a lot in reversing pre-diabetes. You do not need to be all toned and muscled. You merely need to keep the weight that is ideal for your body type, age, and gender. Doing this may also help you *off* from medications if your doctor already prescribes you some.

Opt for fishes and avoid sugar as much as you can, especially the processed ones. Sugar does not only cause you diabetes, but it also creates sluggishness. Also, make your skin look older if you have been bingeing on it. Your body will thank you for the excellent little gestures that you do.

- **Exercise**

Lack of exercise will lead to weight gain and with weight gain on the horizon, the fight to reverse pre-diabetes will soon go out of the window. Weight gain expedites the possibility for you to get actual diabetes so make sure that you get at least a minimum of 15-minute a day exercise to combat this potential.

Exercise may seem like a chore to you, but many people with type 2 diabetes have sworn to this. A day of activity gives so much benefit for you to even pass up on the opportunity to do it while not busy. Your exercise does not need to be strenuous for you to reap its benefits. What matters is including it in your routine and following it religiously.

I know two people personally, one who swears on brisk walking for 30-45 minutes every day and the other one swears on playing table tennis for an hour twice a week. Both people mentioned were diagnosed to be pre-diabetic and are now well away from being actual diabetics. They also do not have to drown themselves on pre-diabetic medications too.

- **Notify your doctor of any changes you notice on your body**

Anything strange that happens to your body must be reported to your doctor. Black or dark spots developing on areas you just scratched on, frequent urinating, wounds that are still fresh and getting infected even after two weeks – those are signs of a person with diabetes, and you have to make sure that your doctor knows if ever anything comes up. This is to help adjust your diet and prescribe you proper medications if needed.

I Just Found Out I Have Diabetes. What Do I Do?

- **Do not panic.**

    I understand this is not an easy feat, considering you just found out that your life is in danger. However, you have to be composed. Do not even think of lingering or taking too much self-pity. It is not going to help you in any way. Keep your composure, cry or share your feelings and fears to a loved one, and slowly pull yourself together. You will need a focused mind and determination.

- **Health plan coverage.**

While your frightened mind is thinking about many things, you will need, what you will feel and many other things that eventually lead to thinking about the unforeseen expenditures for your new-found condition, remind you that there is one thing that needs to be examined first – your health plan. Find out if it covers your condition or not. If included, what are the details? Does it cover medication or specialists? What are the restrictions? If not, find out what needs to be done. This way, you do not have to keep worrying about everything that has to do with your diabetes treatment. Your health plan will be able to provide you more time to worry and enjoy other things despite your new condition.

- **Diet**

   Before signing yourself up for any medication, feel free to go back to your physician and ask if you are still eligible to try reversing it by changing your diet. If yes, find out what kind of diet plans can suit you or better yet, they might be able to point you to the right direction of a good diabetes dietitian who knows the nitty-gritty details of the disease itself. This way, you get to tailor-fit your diet plan well.

   If your condition is way past *just changing your diet plan,* then you may start considering medications. Do not forget to ask what each medicine is for if you are prescribed with more than one.

- **Exercise**

Just because you found out you are sick, does not mean you have to stay in your room and feel depressed or suddenly make the significant change in your lifestyle. Take things a little slow. Of course, I will not ask you to take a pause and smell the flowers, but do not overwhelm yourself. Consider adding exercise to your daily routine because you cannot stay idle if that is how you have been before to being diagnosed. Being idle will only increase your risk of developing advanced diabetes.

Do what you enjoy best. If you are the gym kind of person, consider aerobic, flexibility, or resistance exercises. If not, feel free to enjoy dancing such as Zumba, recreational swimming, brisk walking, yoga, or even martial arts. Exercising does not need to be boring or too official. Keep it fun and incorporate it into your daily routine.

- **Socialize**

Like I said earlier, do not welcome the negative emotions. The situation is already negative enough even to have room for the sad and scary things that your mind creates randomly. Your mind will keep doing that, it is wired to protect you so it will worry as much as it can, but do not swim in the emotions. Just take it to heart that yes, you got your mind's warning and then move on with your life. You are not yet dead, so live and be happy. Communicate with loved ones, communicate with those who have diabetes as well. Find and join a diabetic group if that is what you think you need, but never, ever welcome the negativity.

To feel sad for a while or even cry is just fine. But never go on for days feeling hopeless. This is not the way to live. Share ideas, tips, and even lifehacks with your diabetic community, surely they have some. This will make battling your condition a lot easier.

- **Supplies**

After gathering helpful information from your diabetic community or friends who have experience with diabetes on their own or through a loved one, you may start supplying. Of course, you cannot go to a battle unarmed, so arm yourself with what is needed for your treatment.

One of the most common things that people with diabetes need is the blood glucose meter, lancing device, and test strips. You cannot do without them. Medications and other methods depend on the type of treatment you and your physician have talked about. Make sure consultation comes first before buying your supplies.

- **While at it, explore.**

You may spend some time on finding out more about your condition. There is much information about it all over the internet; there are also books and even programs that can help you explore. Don't just stay in that one dark corner. Find out what you can about diabetes. Treat it like an enemy, find out what it is and find out its weakness. You will find the extra knowledge handy as you go on in life.

- **Schedule**

If you are not the regular kind of person, you will severely need to plot a program that you must follow every day. One thing about diabetes is that it needs to be taken care of in a routine manner. Break that routine, and you might just find yourself wondering when your blood sugar started skyrocketing. Some people will just fall unconscious or crawl to get medical help if they stay clueless with their blood sugar levels for a day or two. Do not wait for this to happen to you.

Plot a schedule that includes your morning monitoring of blood sugar. This lets you determine how you will eat for the rest of the day. Include your medication schedule as well or insulin shots, if you are using this kind of treatment. You cannot forget these things. Set the alarm if you must.

- **Free time**

Last, but not the least, never forget your free time. Again, you are sick, not yet dead. You deserve free time. It is good that you are starting to learn how to manage living while fighting diabetes, but every fighter needs to rest as well. Take a break, enjoy, recuperate, and then once you are well-rested, put your game face on and fight again.

Never forget to spare some free time for your family, loved ones, and yourself. This is what keeps you going, what keeps you sane. Spend quality time with people that love and understand you, enjoy your hobbies and other interests. You are still you; you did not change. It is just that you have to fight quite a big battle, but you should not let that struggle take your personality and dreams away.

Chapter 2: Living with Diabetes

The Diabetic's ABC

A1C

Surely you are familiar with the devices that help you monitor your blood sugar at home, right? They're handy, and they're fast. They do what is expected for it to do – to give you a reading where you can base your food intake or insulin dosage. However, these things are for just that, reading and insulin dosage. It doesn't give you any other details that can help physicians be precise with their treatment approach with your diabetes.

That's where A1C comes in. While your regular blood sugar monitor gives you the general status of your blood sugar, the A1C gives you the percentage of the blood cells in your body that is already wrapped in sugar. Yes, that is what happens to your blood if there's just too much sugar – it becomes your blood's coating. A1C doesn't only help monitor diabetes; it also helps those with prediabetes to know whether their condition is becoming better or worse.

It is to be performed three times a year if you are having a problem controlling your diabetes and twice a year to those who can manage their diabetes well.

Here is your guideline for A1C results:

Percentage	Translation of Blood Sugar Levels
5.7% or less	Normal
5.8 – 6.4%	Elevated / Prediabetes
6.5 % or more	Diabetes

Blood Pressure

As someone with diabetes, you've been monitoring your blood pressure, right? It's for monitoring purposes, so you'd know what is happening to your blood. But why do you want to know what is happening to your blood? What is it for?

Simple. As sugar coats your blood and it passes through your arteries, your arteries get their share of some sugar coating as well – but it happens INSIDE the arteries. In effect, your arteries become narrower, and you become at risk for heart attack and other heart diseases.

And so, what if your arteries becomes narrower, you may think? Think of your regular garden hose. Remember how when you want to play with water as a kid, you block the garden hose's end with your thumb? Then you proceed to open the faucet, so the water comes out of it faster to make that fun splash.

The same principle applies to your blood and arteries. The narrower the passage, the higher the pressure gets for it to pass through your arteries successfully. It's fun with water, but not with your blood. That is something you do not want happening to you. People die, garden hoses do not, and that is precisely why you are monitoring your blood sugar levels.

Blood Pressure	Translation of Blood Pressure
90/60 mmHg* or lower	Hypotension (Low blood pressure)
110/75 mmHg* – 120/80 mmHg*	Normal
120/80 mmHg* – 140/80 mmHg*	Early High Blood Pressure
140/90 mmHg* or higher	Hypertension (High blood pressure)

mmHg (millimeter of mercury) - *a unit of measurement used to determine the amount of pressure.*

Take note that the above indicated is the ideal blood pressure. While most people find it that their blood pressure translation matches easily with the chart above (as surely if you are experiencing hypotension or hypertension, your body WILL let you know), some people do not match this blood pressure translation too. In case your blood pressure translation doesn't match the chart (say for example, at 140/90 mmHg you still feel normal and absolutely no usual signs of hypertension), then I would suggest that you consult your doctor and find out YOUR healthy blood pressure levels. Blood pressure levels may vary with age, weight, lifestyle, and present conditions.

Cholesterol

When you hear the word *cholesterol*, evidently you instantly think that it is terrible. Let me clarify it for you. Cholesterol is a part of your body, apart from the fact that it is also found in foods like dairy, meat, poultry, and seafood. It is an essential component that helps your body digest fat accurately, produce vitamin D, cell membranes, and hormones. Now, that's the right cholesterol you hear about.

There is also the lousy cholesterol also known as LDL or low-density lipoprotein. What does lousy cholesterol do to us?

For one, cholesterol is a substance made of fat. The sad part is that fat does not melt in water, and so, there is no way for it to travel our bloodstream on its own unlike other substances like sugar. Thus, our ever talented bodies thought of binding cholesterol or those fats to some proteins that can travel our bloodstream without any problem. Think of proteins like a cab inside our bodies that offers bloodstream transportation. So, in turn, the cholesterol that is bound to some of our proteins form a combination and *LDL, or bad cholesterol is one of them*.

Once your blood is found to contain a high percentage of this *bad cholesterol*, then it is a sure-fire sign that you are at risk of developing cardiovascular disease. Just imagine all those bad fats being transported and spread evenly to your whole body through your blood.

What do you need to do then? A fasting blood test and a proper diet. This enables you to identify your levels of cholesterol types HDL, LDL, and triglycerides.

You may refer to the chart found on the following page.

The chart contains the data or measurements that is ideal for a person to keep themselves safe from developing diabetes or to prevent it from advancing.

LDL, HDL, and Triglycerides are measured separately. LDL will be measured, and it should not go over 100mg/dl. Anything over the given measurement means danger for you. As for HDL, the analysis should not be any lower than 50mg/dl, or it is heart disease for you. Lastly, with triglycerides, it should be at around 150mg/dl or lower. If it goes higher, you are in for a lifetime of heart disease.

Cholesterol Type	Proper Levels
LDL	100 mg/dl or lower
HDL	50 mg/dl - 70mg/dl or higher to avoid heart disease
Triglycerides	150 mg/dl or lower

*mg/dl - *milligrams per deciliter. Used to measure glucose concentration in the blood.*

Getting On With The Right Nutrition

Seeing as there's just a lot of foods that hide under the bracket of LDL and sugar, how do you eat then? You're not supposed to starve yourself no matter what sickness you have and so, here's what you can eat to survive and enjoy life like you don't have diabetes at all.

- **Dark, Green, Leafy Vegetables (Non-starchy)**

  Vegetables are low in carbs and have few calories, packed with fibers, vitamins, and has proteins as well. Fibers help your digestion, and proteins can give you *a part* of your required protein intake. This means you do not need to stuff yourself with meat every time anymore; you can go for the proper meat servings because of vegetables.

  While most of us love meat, the truth is that it is harder to digest and there's also a big chance that it Is packed with cholesterol in between the meat strands if you were too lazy picking up your grocery. So, go for vegetables in the meantime that you are guilty *because the meat you have in the fridge **isn't** the lean type or worse, the processed type.*

- **Seafood**

Seafood has proteins that are lean and are low in saturated fats. You need to avoid saturated fats at all costs. Enjoy 2-3 servings of fish, especially salmon, every week and you get to have the bonus of absorbing their omega-3 fats as well.

But, what is ***omega-3?***

Officially known as *Omega-3 fatty acids, these* are polyunsaturated fatty acids. By *polyunsaturated,* in layman's term, is the ***healthier version of fat*** that is good for the proper diet as compared to saturated fats.

There are three types of omega-3 fatty acids. One is called **DHA** or docosahexaenoic acid found in fatty fish oils, plant oils called ALA or a-linolenic acid, and the EPA or eicosapentaenoic acid/timnodonic acid also found in fatty fishes like salmon that lives in cold water.

Omega-3 fatty acids keep you safe from developing heart diseases by lowering triglyceride levels if it is elevated. Also, you get to have more benefits from it than just that, especially to those with asthma, depression, and arthritis. So, do not wait to get a result of a high triglyceride level. Enjoy your seafood and keep yourself healthy.

- **Whole Grains**

Forget it if it does not have the word *whole* with it. You need entire grains because any grain that isn't whole is already processed and apart from the fact that the missing nutrients are replaced with sugar, who knows what else is in it? Whole grains help your digestion plus they keep you full longer. However, you have to be careful with the processed ones like your boxed cereals, pasta, white rice, and even the refined white flour.

- **Berries**

Who doesn't like berries? Stuff yourself with these little things. They are packed with antioxidants, manganese, vitamin C, fiber, vitamin K, and potassium. Some of them are sweet, a little sour, but regardless they are all yummy and right for you.

- **Milk & Yogurt**

An excellent source of calcium and most have been fortified to become a good source of Vitamin D; these things contain carbs that are good enough to fill in your daily needs as a person with diabetes. Just make sure to pick one that is low in sugar and fat.

- **Nuts**

One ounce a day is what you need to keep

your hunger at bay. They contain magnesium and fiber, and some even have omega-3 that is undoubtedly good for your heart.

- **Citruses**

Citruses are excellent sources of folate, vitamin C, fiber, and potassium. They make your food zesty, and they fill out your daily vitamin requirements too.

- **Beans**

Go for pinto, black beans, kidney beans, or navy. They are stock full of minerals like potassium and magnesium, they are high in fiber and packed with vitamins too. Half a cup will do just fine for you to give you the right amount of goodies that you need without having to worry about the carbs they contain.

- **Tomatoes**

We knew tomatoes are good for as even as a kid, so what changes that fact? Don't eat them cooked or you'll lose the good stuff. Have them raw to get the most out of the vitamins e and c and the potassium.

- **Stevia**

This is not a part of superfoods, but feel free to enjoy it with your favorite drinks and foods. Stay away from sugar from now on and use stevia instead. It's all-natural and sweet. Have some fun with sweets without feeling guilty.

The Glycemic Index

Another important thing that you need to understand is the glycemic index, especially to those who take insulin. It shows you if there is a rise in your blood glucose levels after two hours that you have consumed a meal that has carbs in it. The measurement or ranking used for the glycemic index is from 0 to 100. Zero being the slowest food to raise your blood glucose levels and 100 being the fastest.

It mostly depends on the content of the food you eat, like the fats, carbohydrates, proteins, and even sodium.

It is used to help you and your doctor to find out how the food you eat reacts to your body and the insulin in it. Though, I have to make it clear that it is not used to measure your production of insulin even if your blood glucose levels rise.

There is no *one size fits all* glycemic index. It varies for every food type and also takes note of the serving size and contents as factors to consider.

So, what is in it for you apart from helping you find out how your body reacts to the food you eat? The glycemic index can help you avoid sudden rise or *spike,* as many people call it, by identifying the foods that are ranked high. The higher glycemic index of the food, the more you should avoid it as it will raise your blood sugar levels in a flash.

Foods that get the glycemic index score of 70 or above is considered high in the index and are mostly composed of foods that are not good for you like processed foods, white bread, pizza, and many other store-bought foods. Foods that score 56 to 69 are considered medium like some fruits that *may* contain natural sugars, some healthier version of your usually unhealthy food like ice cream. The safest glycemic index scores are 55 and less. These include many vegetables like carrots, parsnips, yam, and green peas and fruits like pears, prunes, and apples. It also contains skim milk, whole grain bread, legumes, and beans.

What About Alcohol?

Well, let me make this quick. To those who regularly consume alcohol, also to those who drink more than what their bodies can tolerate, alcohol is not a good idea for people with diabetes, regardless if it is type 1 or type 2. You would not want to dare because there is no such thing as *optimal consumption* for people with diabetes. There is an actual fix, but before we get to that, let me explain the dangers of alcohol consumption for people with diabetes.

The reminder "drink moderately" is not exactly going to cut it anymore for people with diabetes. There is a little exception, but still, it is not as good as it sounds before. You cannot merely drink moderately because doing so will highly likely lead your blood sugar levels to rise.

Remember how almost every alcoholic drinks contain carbohydrates. High levels of carbs, if you do not already know, is highly dangerous for people with diabetes as carbohydrates can cause your blood sugar level to rise dramatically. Even if you say that the alcoholic drink contains 2 to 3 grams of carbs, several bottles will hurt your blood sugar, and you would not want that to happen.

As for heavy drinking, it is dangerous as well. If alcohol moderately raises your blood sugar significantly, heavy drinking, on the other hand, makes your blood sugar *plummet dramatically* into levels that you would not ever dream of going to especially to those who are battling type 1 diabetes.

Deficient blood sugar levels can kill you in minutes. I saw a person, who is battling pre-diabetes experience a superficial blood sugar level, crawl on the floor, covered in cold sweat, and does not even know if she would vomit first or take care of her seemingly uncontrollable bowel movement. It is frightening to witness.

In such an occasion, the person **must be** given medical attention **as soon as possible;** there is no room for delay in any manner. A delay will lead to that person's death so fast you would not know what hit you.

Going back to the topic, avoid alcohol as much as you can, especially sweet wine and beer. Rum, gin, vodka, and whiskey are also some drinks to prevent as they lead to the massive drop in sugar levels.

You may enjoy liquor once in a while but avoid the mixers as they have tons of sugar in them. Also, make sure that the alcohol you intend to enjoy is carbohydrate-free. If you want to be extra safe, you may add seltzer or water to your drink as well. Wines are also excellent, especially for the heart, just make sure they are not sweetened. And as always, do not go wasted.

Don't You Dare Forget About the Routine Care

Everyone has to have their daily routine, either that or you risk messing up your whole day including eating and sleeping patterns. That goes for people with diabetes too. Treat it like this, if your body has been aching some time and sending you pain signals, it is begging for you to take care of it better than before. And what better way to repay the vessel that enables you to enjoy life with your family than setting up a healthy routine for it?

1. Monitor

Monitoring frequency depends on what your doctor tells you, but the best time to start is in the morning. This enables you how to plan your meals for the rest of the day and before you take your insulin shots if you are to have them. It seems quite a job in the first few weeks, but you'll warm up to it and realize its importance soon enough.

2. Manage

It is a bit like sailing, without a heading (monitoring your sugar), you pretty much do not know where to go. As soon as you're done with monitoring and are used to your blood sugar's fluctuations, then you can refine the diet that was initially prescribed to you. Do not be overwhelmed if you are asked to change your diet. It's all for you and as soon as you are familiar with it and its effects on your body, you can make some adjustments to customize it further for your needs with the help of your doctor.

3. Stick

Stick to your medications especially the schedule. They are there for a reason and not taking them, well, defeats just that very purpose. Missing one plan of medicine intake can undo your hard work of maintaining your diet. Don't let it happen. Might as well keep a pillbox and put a magnet on it, stick it in your fridge. That way, you do not forget it.

4. Exercise

When I say training, walking will do. You do not need to weight the heavy stuff just to make a point to your body that you are, in fact, trying to keep it in shape. Keeping in shape is only secondary, it's your heart that we are trying to protect her. Make sure it stays active, and you burn what needs burning while you walk and enjoy that time of the day when it is most convenient for you.

What Is the Right Treatment for You

You are not one to decide it on your own. Once you are diagnosed with diabetes, you can't go all DIY on it. I'm not saying either that you should be too dependent on your doctor. It needs collaboration to figure out what is truly good for you. Inform your doctor what your body shows you and what your body's reactions are to certain medications and food, your doctor decides the dosages and frequencies, and you agree to settle for the right treatment.

This doesn't stop the first time you get diagnosed. As your body adjusts to medications and copes with age, your body will respond to previous drugs it wasn't okay with before and stop responding to medications you are used to. So, adjustment, acceptance, and cooperation are the key.

Diet + Exercise

Diet AND exercise is one type of treatment for diabetics, especially if newly diagnosed and the status of diabetes is not that serious. However, for diet and exercise, you have to understand that one cannot go without the other, they always have to be together to fortify the protection that you build for your body by controlling what you put in it and how you maintain it. Also, dieting for your diabetes should be tailor-fit for your needs. It's not like a ready-made t-shirt that you can just grab from a stand and try on. YOUR DIET SHOULD ALWAYS GO WITH YOUR AGE, WEIGHT, LIFESTYLE, and CURRENT CONDITIONS – no more, no less.

As for exercise, there's no need for you to go all out on it primarily if you are not used to strenuous activities. Walking or brisk walking with your loved one and your dog, doing yoga or your favorite martial arts, and even recreational swimming will do. Just make sure to do it every day for about 30, minutes, and you will do just fine.

Oral Medication

Oral Medication is the option when diet and exercise are not cutting it for you anymore. Some of these medications are to encourage your liver not to dispose of all the glucose that passes through it, some are meant to help prevent your pancreas from breaking down the hormones that help produce insulin, and some encourage your pancreas to produce more insulin.

There are many other medications for diabetes that will help you out directly, however, again this needs the go signal of your doctor if you are to start any of these medicines.

Injectables

Just because you see a diabetic injecting medication does not mean it is already insulin. It's not always insulin. At times, there are medications that people with diabetes need to help them slow down their digestion. To prevent them from frequently eating to improve their livers by slowing down the glucose production. Just like oral medication, there is a myriad of function for injectable medicines meant for people with diabetes. Again, this depends on your doctor's findings and suggestions.

Insulin

Not all diabetics need insulin injections or pumps. Those people with diabetes type 1 need insulin, but not always for those with diabetes type 2. Insulin is to be taken ONLY if your blood sugar is getting more and more difficult to control. There are other methods to get insulin into your body, and that is through injection, inhaler, through insulin pen, and even insulin pumps.

Weight Loss Surgery

If none of the above is cutting it anymore for you and your doctor thinks that in your current state, having a weight loss surgery is the best option, then go for it. Please be advised that weight loss surgery is not for everyone and some people have to make do with the above options.

Weight loss surgery will, like the name says, a slash of a right amount of your weight and make controlling of your blood sugar a lot easier than it did before. As an effect, it increases the hormones *incretins* responsible for your pancreas' insulin production. It has a lot of benefits. But do not opt for this if your diabetes is still controllable with a combination of the above treatments unless you are overweight and your blood sugar is really out of control.

Chapter 3: Creating a Life-Changing Action Plan

Know Your Treatment Goals

What do you think is your ultimate treatment goal? Yes, that is to keep your blood sugar ALWAYS, ALWAYS, at bay. However, that is not as easy as you can say it. And so, you have to know it, remember it, and live with it.

Another thing that you have to add to your goal is to prevent tissue damage from happening to you because of too much sugar that flows into your bloodstream.

Since you already know your targets for healthy blood sugar by basing on the previous chapter, all you have to do is not to forget monitoring your blood sugar. When your schedule for an A1C test arrives, do not, AT ALL COST, skip it. Treat it as something significant because getting the results from that analysis will let you know if there have been good or bad changes in your diabetes. Surely, you do not want to keep to a diet that does not fit you anymore, right?

Identifying the Steps to Take

The following are your regular *must-do*, every time you visit your doctor.

1. Monitor Your Blood Glucose

I know you have repeatedly been told to monitor your blood glucose so you'd know how to work on it as your day pans out. And I am repeating it now because your life depends on it, no kidding. So, wherever you go, may it be your house or the hospital, don't ever miss it.

2. Get Your Blood Pressure Monitored

The next most important thing after your blood sugar is your blood pressure. If you keep monitoring one without the other, then the purpose of your treatment is lost. Blood sugar and blood pressure go hand in hand because it involves both your blood and heart.

3. Check Your Foot

What's the foot got to do with your diabetes? Well, your feet are like the window to your diabetic body. Anything that goes exceptionally wrong with your blood circulation and even damage to your nerves will inevitably show through your feet. The same principle applies to diabetes and infections.

4. Check Your Weight

Your weight, apart from your feet, says a lot about your diet. It's not always an identifier of diabetes, *but* checking your blood glucose as soon as your weight rises is the best way of protecting yourself not only from diabetes but also heart diseases.

5. Review Your Treatment Plan

Always, always review your treatment plan with your doctor before you leave the hospital. You need to let your doctor know of any changes in your body's reaction to your current medication and diet as this *may* mean having to change your doses, medicine, and even your dietary plan.

6. A1C Test

Don't forget your A1C test as well. This analysis should be performed twice to thrice a year depending on the levels of your diabetes.

Tracking Your Progress

Why should you track your progress? Tracking your progress can help your physician more than you can imagine as your journal will contain details of your daily life as you try your best (and sometimes failing) to control your blood sugar and your diabetes in general.

Make sure to track:

- Weight gain

- Weight losses

- Eating habits

- Eating behaviours

- Daily blood sugar results

Be as honest as you can and do not ever think that you are doing it for your doctor. You are doing it for yourself to help you become better and to be successful in fighting your diabetes. If you are not as comfortable using a physical journal, there are numerous apps found on the internet that is made for diabetes alone. However, the problem with keeping your progress through an app is your battery's availability.

Still, go for one which makes you feel most comfortable. After all, the most important thing here is what can be found in your diabetes journal.

Chapter 4: The Healing Diet

To help you out with your battle with diabetes, let us not only stick with words of advice, steps to follow, tips, and encouragements. Let me spare a whole chapter for some yummy recipes that won't make you worry about your blood sugar.

7 Smoothie Recipe

Raspberry and Peanut Butter Smoothie

Serves: 2

Preparation: 10 minutes

Ingredients:

- Peanut butter, smooth and natural [2 tbsp]
- Skim milk [2 tbsp]
- Raspberries, fresh [1 or 1 ½ cups]

- Ice cubes [1 cup]

- Stevia [2 tsp]

Directions:

Put in all the ingredients in your blender. Set the mixer to puree, wait until smooth. Serve. Good for 2.

Calories	Fat	Carbs	Protein	Sodium
170	8.6g	20g	5.1g	67mg

Strawberry, Kale and Ginger Smoothie

Serves: 2

Preparation: 10 minutes

Ingredients:

- Curly kale leaves, fresh and large with stems removed [6 pcs]

- Grated ginger, raw and peeled [2 tsp]

- Water, cold [½ cup]

- Lime juice [3 tbsp]

- Honey [2 tsp]

- Strawberries, fresh and trimmed [1 or 1 ½ cups]

- Ice cubes [1 cup]

Directions:

Put in all the ingredients in your blender. Set the mixer to puree, wait until smooth. Serve. Good for 2.

Calories	Fat	Carbohydrates	Protein	Sodium
205	2.9g	42.4g	4.2g	0.083 mg

Almond + Blueberry Smoothie

Serves: 2

Preparation: 10 minutes

Ingredients:

- Almonds, slivered [1/4 cup]

- Stevia [2 tsp]

- Wheat germ [2 tbsp]

- Blueberries, fresh [1 or 1 ½ cups]

- Greek yogurt [½ cup]

- Ice cube [1 cup]

- Almond or skim milk, unsweetened [2 tbsp]

Directions:

Put in all the ingredients in your blender. Set the mixer to puree, wait until smooth. Serve. Good for 2.

Calories	Fat	Carbohydrates	Protein	Sodium
225	8g	31g	11.4g	34mg

Cottage Cheese and Spiced Raspberry Smoothie

Serves: 2

Preparation: 10 minutes

Ingredients:

- Rolled oats, old-fashioned [2 tbsp]

- Cottage cheese, fat-free [½ cup]

- Dates pitted [2 pcs.]

- Stevia [1 tsp]

- Ice cubes [1 cup]

- Cinnamon, ground [1 pinch]

- Fresh raspberries, [1 ½ cups]

Directions:

Put in all the ingredients in your blender. Set the blender to puree, wait until smooth. Serve. Good for 2.

Calories	Fat	Carbohydrates	Protein	Sodium
134	1g	25g	8.4g	216mg

Flax Seed and Strawberry-Banana Smoothie

Serves: 2

Preparation: 10 minutes

Ingredients:

- Stevia [2 tsp]

- Skim milk [2 tbsp]

- Flaxseed, ground [2 tbsp]

- Tofu, soft [½ cup]

- Banana, medium-sized [sliced]

- Ice cubes [1 cup]

- Strawberries, fresh and trimmed [1 or 1 ½ cups]

Directions:

Put in all the ingredients in your blender. Set the blender to puree, wait until smooth. Serve. Good for 2.

Calories	Fat	Carbohydrates	Protein	Sodium
159	4.7g	25g	7.7g	10mg

Green Apple and Spinach Smoothie

Serves: 2

Preparation: 10 minutes

Ingredients:

- Stevia [2 tsp]

- Ice cube [1 cup]

- Greek yogurt [½ cup]

- Apple or orange juice, unsweetened [1/3 cup]

- Small apple, chopped and cored [1 pc]

- Stevia [1 tsp]

- Flax seeds. Ground [2 tbsp]

- Baby Spinach [2 cups]

Directions:

Put in all the ingredients in your blender. Set the blender to puree, wait until smooth. Serve. Good for 2.

Calories	Fat	Carbohydrates	Protein	Sodium
138	2.4g	24g	7.4g	69mg

Blackberry and Nuts Smoothie

Serves: 2

Preparation: 10 minutes

Ingredients:

- Stevia [2 tsp]

- Greek yogurt [½ cup]

- Ice cubes [1 cup]

- Almond butter [2 tbsp]

- Blackberries, fresh [1 or ½ cup]

Directions:

Put in all the ingredients in your blender. Set the blender to puree, wait until smooth. Serve. Good for 2.

Calories	Fat	Carbohydrates	Protein	Sodium
175	9.3g	16g	9.6g	57mg

Green Smoothies

Green Diabetic Smoothie

Serves: 2

Preparation: 10 minutes

Ingredients:

- Orange, large [1 pc]

- Kale [1 cup]

- Spinach [2 cups]

- Celery [3 stalks]

- Cucumber, large [1 pc]

- Ice cubes [1 cup]

Directions:

Put in all the ingredients in your blender. Set the blender to puree, wait until smooth. Serve. Good for 2.

Calories	Fat	Carbohydrates	Protein	Sodium
250	1g	30g	8g	0mg

Delectable Sweet Potato Smoothie

Serves: 2

Preparation: 10 minutes

Ingredients:

- Orange, large [1 pc]

- Sweet potato, cooked and peeled [½ cup]

- Banana, frozen [½ cup]

- Cinnamon [¼ tsp]

- Almond milk, unsweetened [1/2 cup]

- Almond butter [1 tbsp]

Directions:

Put in all the ingredients in your blender. Set the blender to puree, wait until smooth. Enjoy.

Calories	Fat	Carbohydrates	Protein	Sodium
262.5	4.9g	50.4g	4.6g	417.6mg

Very Berry Smoothie

Serves: 2

Preparation: 10 minutes

Ingredients:

- Kale [3 pcs]

- Mango chunks, fresh [a handful]

- Blueberries, frozen [1 cup]

- Flax meal [2 tbsp]

- Blackberries, frozen [1 cup]

- Pure coconut water, unsweetened [2 cups]

Directions:

Put in all the ingredients in your blender. Set the blender to puree, wait until smooth. Enjoy.

Calories	Fat	Carbohydrates	Protein	Sodium
148	0g	35g	2g	25mg

Green, Green, Green

Serves: 2

Preparation: 10 minutes

Ingredients:

- Ginger, peeled and sliced [1 cm]

- Celery, cut into chunks [½ stick]

- Mint leaves [12 pcs]

- Cucumber, cut into thick slices [2 inches]

- Baby spinach [a handful]

- Cold press apple juice [1 ¼ cup]

Directions:

Put in all the ingredients in your blender. Set the blender to puree, wait until smooth. Enjoy.

Calories	Fat	Carbohydrates	Protein	Sodium
250	1g	33.4g	8g	0mg

Spinach, Chia Seed, and Coco Smoothie

Serves: 2

Preparation: 10 minutes

Ingredients:

- Ginger, peeled and sliced [1 cm]

- Celery, cut into chunks [½ stick]

- Mint leaves [12 pcs]

- Cucumber, cut into thick slices [2 inches]

- Baby spinach [a handful]

- Cold press apple juice [1 ¼ cup]

Directions:

Put in all the ingredients in your blender. Set the blender to puree, wait until smooth. Enjoy.

Calories	Fat	Carbohydrates	Protein	Sodium
354	4g	58g	22g	0.083 mg

Go Nutty-Berry Smoothie

Serves: 2

Preparation: 10 minutes

Ingredients:

- Ginger, peeled and sliced [1 cm]

- Chia seeds [2 tsp]

- Cinnamon [½ tsp]

- Almond butter [1 tbsp]

- Banana, frozen [½ a piece]

- Mixed berries, frozen [½ cup]

- Stevia [1 tsp]

- Almond milk [1 cup]

- Flaxseed, ground [1 tbsp]

Directions:

Put in all the ingredients in your blender. Set the blender to puree, wait until smooth. Enjoy.

Calories	Fat	Carbohydrates	Protein	Sodium
154.6	7.7g	21.3g	3.2g	91.6mg

Yummy Oatmeal Berry Smoothie

Serves: 2

Preparation: 10 minutes

Ingredients:

- Old fashioned rolled oats [½ cup]

- Vanilla yogurt or Greek yogurt [⅓ cup]

- Frozen berries [½ cup]

- Ice cube [1 cup]

- Milk [1 cup]

- Stevia [2 tbsp]

Directions:

Put in all the ingredients in your blender. Set the blender to puree, wait until smooth. Enjoy.

Calories	Fat	Carbohydrates	Protein	Sodium
177	1g	32g	11g	20mg

7 - Chicken Recipes Ideal for Lunch and Dinner

Chicken Parmesan Drumstick: Finger-Licking Good Without the Guilt

Serves: 3-4

Ingredients:

- Paprika [1 tsp]

- Dried oregano, crushed [2 tsp]

- Lemon wedges

- Eggs, beaten [2 pcs]

- Black pepper [¼ tsp]

- Butter melted [¼ cup]

- Snipped fresh oregano

- Fine dry bread crumbs [¾ cup]

- Grated Parmesan cheese [¾ cup]

- Chicken drumsticks skinned [16 pcs]

- Fat-free milk [¼ cup]

Directions:

Set oven to 375 deg. F. Line, foil, and grease two shallow and large baking pans. Set aside. Combine egg and milk in a small bowl. In another shallow dish, add bread crumbs, paprika, oregano, parmesan, and pepper. Dip the drumsticks into the egg mixture and then coat with the crumbs.

Place drumsticks in pans and drizzle with butter. Bake for 45 – 50 mins while uncovered. Wait for the chicken to become tender. Sprinkle with oregano and add lemon wedges for garnishing.

Calories	Fat	Carbohydrates	Protein	Sodium
336	4g	38g	38g	532mg

Buffalo-Style Chicken Salad: A Hint of Spice to Tickle Your Palate

Serves: 2

Ingredients:

- Paprika [1 tsp]
- Fat-free blue cheese salad dressing [1 tbsp]
- Cracked black pepper [1/4 tsp]
- Cooked chicken breast, chopped [3/4 cup]
- Fat-free milk [1 tsp]
- Celery, cut into sticks [1 pc]
- Buffalo wing sauce [2 tbsp]
- Light blue cheese, crumbled
- Heart of romaine sliced [Half]

Directions:

Place the romaine in a bowl. Place chopped chicken and sauce in a microwave-safe bowl.

Microwave the diced chicken and sauce on high for a minute. Add the microwaved mixture over the romaine. Add cheese and pepper for toppings. Combine milk and salad dressing and then drizzle over your salad. Add celery sticks and serve.

Calories	Fat	Carbohydrates	Protein	Sodium
297	10g	13g	37g	596mg

Louisiana Chicken: The Ultimate Companion for your Day or Night Meal

Serves: 2-3

Ingredients:

- Frozen cut okra [1 cup]

- Black pepper [1 tsp]

- Stewed tomatoes, no salt [1 can]

- Skinned drumsticks [8 pcs]

- Louisiana hot sauce [1 ½ tbsp.]

- Whole grain noodles, cooked [2 cups]

- Dried thyme, ground [1 tsp]

- Salt [1/4 tsp]

Directions:

Coat a skillet lightly with cooking spray. Place it over medium-high heat and add chicken. Let it turn brown on all sides and don't forget to set them. Add stewed tomatoes on top, thyme, hot sauce, okra, pepper, and salt. Let it boil and then reduce the heat. Cover and then simmer until the center is no longer pink. Add the chicken on a platter and then the sauce. Serve with the noodles and enjoy.

Calories	Fat	Carbohydrates	Protein	Sodium
190	1g	8g	27g	500mg

Thai Chicken Wings: A Quick Fix For Your Exotic Dish Craving

Serves: 7-8

Ingredients:

- Lime juice [1 tbsp]

- Ground ginger [1/4 tsp]

- Peanut Sauce

- Chicken wing drummettes [24 pcs]

- Water [1/4 cup]

- Crushed red pepper [1/4 tsp]

- Garlic, minced [2 cloves]

- Water [1/2 cup]

- Reduced-sodium soy sauce [2 tsp]

- Almond butter [1/2 cup]

- Ground ginger [1/2 tsp]

Directions:

Put chicken in the slow cooker. Add the lime juice, water, and ginger. Cover and set to low heat. Let it cook for 5-6 hrs. Drain the chicken and discard the liquid. Add half of the peanut sauce to chicken and toss. Serve.

Calories	Fat	Carbohydrates	Protein	Sodium
101	1g	3g	9g	159mg

Chicken Mac & Cheese: Diabetic-Friendly and Just Super Yummy

Serves: 2

Ingredients:

- Finely chopped onion [1/4 cup]

- Dried multigrain [1 ½ cups]

- Fresh baby spinach [2 cups]

- Skinless, boneless chicken breast halves, cut into 1-inch pieces [12 oz]

- Fat-free milk [1 2/3 cups]

- Chopped, seeded tomatoes [1 cup]

- All-purpose flour [1 tbsp]

- Shredded reduced-fat cheddar cheese [3/4 cup]

- Light semi soft cheese with garlic and herb [[1 6 1/2 oz]

Directions:

Cook the macaroni in a saucepan. Make sure to follow package directions. Don't add salt. Drain the macaroni. Coat a skillet with cooking spray. Heat the skillet over medium-high heat. Add the chicken and onions. Let it cook until onion is transparent and chicken is no longer pink. Stir frequently. Remove the skillet from heat. Add the cheese until it melts. Whisk flour and milk in another bowl. Add the chicken mixture. Cook over medium-high heat and stir. Wait until thick and bubbly then reduce the heat to low. Add the macaroni until heated. Add tomatoes and spinach. Serve.

Calories	Fat	Carbohydrates	Protein	Sodium
169	3g	24g	11g	210mg

Five Spice Chicken Wings: Put Your Fingers and

Serves: 4-5

Ingredients:

- Finely chopped onion [1/4 cup]

- Plum sauce [3/4 cup]

- Five-spice powder [1 tsp]

- Butter melted [1 tbsp]

- Slivered green onions

- Chicken wings [16 pcs]

Directions:

Preheat your oven to 375 deg. F. Cut off the tips of the wings and discard the tips. Cut each wing into two pieces. Line a baking pan with foil and arrange the wings in it in a single layer. Bake the wings for 20 minutes. Drain. In a slow cooker, add the butter, five spice powder, plum sauce and chicken. Stir to coat the chicken with sauce.

Cover and cook on low heat. Do this for 4 hours.

Serve.

Calories	Fat	Carbohydrates	Protein	Sodium
32	1g	3g	3g	45mg

Balsamic and Dijon Chicken: Your Ultimate Grilled Chicken Craving Buster

Serves: 2

Ingredients:

*   Balsamic vinegar [3 tbsp]

*   Snipped fresh thyme [2 tsp]

*   Dijon-style mustard [1/3 cup]

*   Garlic, minced [2 cloves]

*   Skinless, boneless chicken breast halves [4 pcs]

*   Fresh thyme sprigs

Directions:

In a resealable plastic bag placed over a shallow dish, add the chicken and set aside. Prepare the marinade by stirring the balsamic vinegar, mustard, thyme, and garlic until smooth. Pour the marinade on the chicken inside the plastic and seal the bag. Turn bag to coat the chicken and leave in the fridge for 24 hours. Turn the bag if needed. Drain the chicken, don't discard the marinade. Place the chicken on the grill directly over coals. Grill, the chicken for 7 minutes and brush with marinade. Turn the chicken and coat again with marinade. Garnish with thyme sprigs. Serve.

Calories	Fat	Carbohydrates	Protein	Sodium
161	1g	3g	26g	537mg

7 - Pork Recipes Ideal for Lunch and Dinner

Quick Pork Diane: Delectable Dish Under 30 Minutes

Serves: 4

Ingredients:

- Lemon juice [1 tsp]

- Snipped fresh chives, parsley, or oregano [1 tbsp]

- Water [1 tbsp]

- Dijon-style mustard [1 tsp]

- Butter [1 tbsp]

- Worcestershire sauce [1 tbsp]

- Lemon-pepper seasoning [1 tsp]

- Four boneless pork top loin chops

Directions:

To make the sauce, add water, lemon juice, mustard, and Worcestershire sauce in a bowl and set aside. Remove the fat from the chops and sprinkle each side with lemon-pepper seasoning. Melt butter in a skillet and add the chops. Cook for 12 minutes and turn to cook the other side. Remove from heat. Transfer to serving platter and cover with foil. Pour the sauce into the skillet and then pour the sauce over the chops. Top the chops with chives. Serve.

Calories	Fat	Carbohydrates	Protein	Sodium
178	11g	1g	18g	302mg

Mediterranean Pork Chops: A 5-Ingredient Dish You Wouldn't Want to Miss

Serves: 1

Ingredients:

- Boneless or bone-in pork loin chops cut 1/2 inch thick (1 pc)
- Salt [1/4 tsp]
- Freshly ground black pepper [1/4 tsp]
- Finely snipped fresh rosemary or 1 tsp dried rosemary, crushed [1 tbsp]
- Garlic, minced [3 cloves]

Directions:

Prepare the oven by preheating to 425 deg. F. Line a roasting pan with foil and sprinkle the chops with salt and pepper. Set aside. Add rosemary and garlic, combine in a bowl. Sprinkle them evenly on the chops. Place the chops in the pan. Roast for 10 minutes. Reduce the oven temp to 350 deg. F and serve.

Calories	Fat	Carbohydrates	Protein	Sodium
161	5g	1g	25g	192mg

Spicy Grilled Portlets: Perfect Dish For Adventurous Eaters

Serves: 3-4

Ingredients:

- Sliced mango or chili peppers

- Lime juice [¼ cup]

- Olive oil [1 tbsp]

- Salt [¼ tsp]

- Garlic, minced [2 cloves]

- Ground cinnamon [1 tsp]

- Chili powder [1 tbsp]

- Ground cumin [2 tsp]

- Hot pepper sauce [½ tsp]

- Four pork rib chops, cut ¾ inch thick

Directions:

Place the chops in a plastic bag. To make the marinade, add chili powder, lime juice, cumin, oil, cinnamon, garlic, hot pepper, and salt. Pour them over the chops and seal the bag. Turn the bag to coat chops well. Place the chops in the fridge for 24 hours. Make sure to turn the bag to even out the marinade. Drain the chops and discard the marinade. Grill the chops until pork juices run clear. Turn once. Garnish with mango or chili peppers. Serve.

Calories	Fat	Carbohydrates	Protein	Sodium
196	9g	3g	25g	159mg

Tender Pork in Mushroom Sauce: That Perfect Comfort Dish For Every Occasion

Serves: 4

Ingredients:

- Cooking oil [1 tbsp]
- Worcestershire sauce [1½ tsp]
- Dried thyme, crushed [¾ tsp]
- 1 (10.75 ounces) can reduced-fat, reduced-sodium condensed cream of mushroom soup
- Pork loin chops, cut ¾ inch thick (4 pcs)
- Garlic powder [1 tsp]
- Apple juice or apple cider [½ cup]
- One small onion, thinly sliced
- Sliced fresh mushrooms [1½ cups]
- Fresh thyme sprigs
- Quick-cooking tapioca [2 tbsp]

Directions:

Remove the fat from the chops. Place a skillet over medium heat and add oil then warm. Add the chops and cook until brown. Drain the fat. Add the onion in a slow cooker and add the chops. Crush the tapioca and add it to a bowl together with Worcestershire sauce, thyme, garlic powder, apple juice, mushrooms and mushroom soup. Pour the mixture over the chops. Cover the slow cooker and cook on low heat for 8 to 9 hours. Garnished with thyme sprigs. Serve.

Calories	Fat	Carbohydrates	Protein	Sodium
152	2g	4g	26g	286mg

Pork and Herb-Tomato Sauce: A Slow-Cooked Dish Perfect For the Family

Serves: 4

Ingredients:

- Quick-cooking tapioca crushed [2 tsp]

- Salt [¼ tsp]

- Worcestershire sauce [½ tsp]

- Minced garlic (3 cloves)

- Four pork rib chops (with bone), cut ¾ inch thick

- Small onion, chopped [1 pc]

- Stewed tomatoes, undrained and unsalted [2 cans]

- Crushed red pepper [1/4 tsp]

- Ground black pepper [½ tsp]

- Dried Italian seasoning, crushed [1 tsp]

Directions:

Remove the fat from the chops and lightly coat the skillet with cooking spray. Place skillet over medium-high heat. Cook the chops until brown on both sides and set aside. In a slow cooker, add the garlic, onion, tapioca, black pepper, Italian seasoning, crushed red pepper, Worcestershire sauce, and salt. Add the chops and pour the tomatoes. Cover the slow cooker and cook on low heat for 8 hours. Transfer the chops to a platter, add tomatoes on top and serve.

Calories	Fat	Carbohydrates	Protein	Sodium
245	7g	19g	24g	568mg

Cranberry Pork Loin: Sweet and Tangy, Perfect For the Tummy

Serves: 4

Ingredients:

- Cooking oil [1 tbsp]
- Honey [1 tbsp]
- Salt [1/8 tsp]
- Ground nutmeg [1/8 tsp]
- Ground black pepper [1/8 tsp]
- Frozen orange juice concentrate, thawed [2 tbsp]
- Ground ginger [¼ tsp]
- Whole cranberry sauce [½ cup]
- 4 (5 ounces) boneless pork loin chops, cut ½-inch thick

Directions:

Coat a skillet with nonstick cooking spray and place over medium-high heat. Sprinkle salt and pepper on both sides of chops and put it on the skillet. Reduce the heat to medium and let the chops cook until done. Make sure you turn the chops. Remove the chops from the skillet and cover with foil. Add orange juice concentrate, honey, nutmeg, ginger, and cranberry sauce in a bowl and mix. Add the mixture to the skillet and cook for 2 minutes until sauce thickens. Pour over the chops and serve.

Calories	Fat	Carbohydrates	Protein	Sodium
277	9g	22g	26g	288mg

Sassy Pork Chops: Quick and Easy, Delectable and Yummy

Serves: 2

Ingredients:

- Ground black pepper [1/4 tsp]
- Reduced-sodium chicken broth [1/4 cup]
- Dried oregano, crushed [1/2 tsp]
- Orange juice [1/4 cup]
- Cooking oil [2 tbsp]
- Chopped onion [1/2 cup]
- Eight pork loin chops (with bone), cut 3/4 inch thick
- Medium red, green, and sweet yellow peppers cut into strips [2 pcs]
- Garlic salt [1/2 tsp]
- Thinly sliced celery [1 cup]

- Chopped chipotle chili peppers in adobo sauce [1 tbsp]

Directions:

In a slow cooker, add the celery, onion, and sweet peppers. Set aside. Season the chops with salt and pepper. Place in the skillet and cook over medium heat until brown on both sides. Add the chops to the cooker. Add broth, chipotle peppers, orange juice, and oregano in a bowl. Mix and pour on the chops. Cover the cooker and place the low heat. Cook for 7 hours. Place the chops and veggies on a platter and discard the liquid before serving.

Calories	Fat	Carbohydrates	Protein	Sodium
215	7g	4g	33g	363mg

7 - Beef Recipes Ideal for Lunch and Dinner

Beef and Broccoli: A Classic All-Hit Dish

Serves: 2

Ingredients:

- Hoisin sauce [3 tbsp]

- Cornstarch [3 tsp]

- Reduced-sodium soy sauce [1 tbsp]

- Garlic, minced [3 cloves]

- Boneless beef top sirloin steak, bias-sliced 1/8-inch thick* [12 oz]

- Reduced-sodium beef broth [3/4 cup]

- Toasted sesame oil [2 tsp]

- Canola oil [1 tbsp]

- Crushed red pepper [1/4 tsp]

- Water [2 tbsp]

- Quartered and halved cherry tomatoes [1 cup]
- Chinese egg noodles or whole wheat vermicelli [4 oz]
- Fresh broccoli [1 lb]

Directions:

Add 2 tsp. Cornstarch, garlic, red pepper, and soy sauce in a bowl and mix. Add the beef and coat with the mixture. Set aside and marinate for 20 minutes. Cook the noodles based on the instructions in the package and do not add salt. Set aside when done. Cut the broccoli into 2 inches, peel and set apart. Prepare the sauce by adding water, hoisin sauce, sesame oil and one tsp cornstarch. Set aside. Heat the oil over medium-high heat in a skillet. Add the beef mixture and stir-fry for 2 minutes until you see the center become less pink. Remove from heat and set aside. Add the beef broth to the skillet and then the broccoli. Let it boil and reduce the heat to medium. Cover the skillet and cook until the broccoli is tender. Add the sauce to the broccoli, cook and stir until it thickens. Add the beef and tomatoes, heat them for a while and serve over the noodles.

Calories	Fat	Carbohydrates	Protein	Sodium
379	14g	39g	26g	532mg

Greek Feta Burgers: Who Says You Can't Indulge in Burgers?

Serves: 1

Ingredients:

- Ground black pepper [1/4 tsp]
- Snipped fresh flat-leaf parsley [1 1/2 tsp]
- Fresh spinach leaves [1/2 cup]
- Crumbled reduced-fat feta cheese [1 tbsp]
- Garlic, minced [1 clove]
- One whole wheat hamburger bun, split and toasted
- Cucumber Sauce
- 90 percent or higher lean ground beef [8 oz]
- Tomato slices [2 pcs]
- Thin slivers red onion
- Ground black pepper [1/8 tsp]

Directions:

Prepare the cucumber sauce and set aside. Combine the cheese, garlic, parsley, ground beef, and pepper in a bowl. Mix and shape into 2-inch thick patties. Cook the patties in a skillet over medium-high heat for about 10 minutes and turn to cook the other side evenly. Line the bun halves with spinach and top it with tomato slices, patties, and sauce. Garnish with red onion and serve.

Calories	Fat	Carbohydrates	Protein	Sodium
292	14g	14g	27g	356mg

Grilled Flank Steak Salad: One Recipe You'd Be Glad About

Serves: 1

Ingredients:

- Cherry tomatoes halved [4 pcs]
- Small yellow and red sweet peppers, stemmed, seeded, and halved [2 pcs]
- Small avocado, halved, seeded, peeled, and thinly sliced [1/4]
- Green onions trimmed [2 pcs]
- Cilantro Dressing
- Torn romaine lettuce [2 cups]
- Fresh cilantro sprigs
- Fresh corn, husked and silks removed [1 ear]
- Beef flank steak [8 oz]

Directions:

Divide the dressing into 2 portions then remove the fat from the steak. Score both sides of the steak in a diamond pattern by cutting shallow diagonals at 1-inch distances. Place the steak in a resealable plastic bag and pour the other half of the cilantro dressing. Seal the bag and set aside the remaining dressing. Turn the bag to coat the steak and marinate for 30 mins in the fridge. Coat the corn, sweet pepper, and green onions with cooking spray. Grill the steak and corn on the griller until the steak is cooked as desired and the corn is tender. Turn the steak once to cook both sides evenly. Reduce the heat to medium and add the meat, followed by the veggies after a couple of minutes, on the griller. Cover and then grill. Slice the meat against the grain and chop the sweet peppers and onions.

Cut the corn from the cob and leave the kernels in sheets. Serve the meat, veggies, and tomatoes over the lettuce. Drizzle it with the remaining dressing and garnish with cilantro sprigs.

Calories	Fat	Carbohydrates	Protein	Sodium
357	15g	31g	29g	376mg

Super Loaded Nachos: Top-Notch Dish Perfect For Sharing

Serves: 1

Ingredients:

- Homemade Taco Seasoning
- Ground turmeric [1/4 tsp]
- Shredded reduced-fat cheddar cheese [1/2 cup]
- Paprika [1/4 tsp]
- All-purpose flour [1 tbsp]
- Extra-lean ground beef [8 oz]
- Shredded part-skim mozzarella cheese [1/2 cup]
- Eight 6-inch corn tortillas
- Fat-free cream cheese, softened [1 oz]
- Fat-free milk [3/4 cup]
- Unsalted butter [2 tsp]

- Water [1/4 cup]

- Sliced green onions [1/4 cup]

- Chopped tomato [1 cup]

- Fresh jalapeno chile pepper, stemmed, seeded, and thinly sliced [1 pc]

- Snipped fresh cilantro [2 tbsp]

- Chopped green or red sweet pepper [1/2 cup]

- Chunky mild salsa [1/2 cup]

Directions:

Heat the oven to 375 deg. F and line the baking sheet with parchment paper. Cut the tortilla into eight wedges and place it in a single layer on the baking sheet. Coat the wedges with cooking spray and bake until wedges become crisp and golden brown. Set aside. To make the cheese sauce, melt the butter in a saucepan over medium heat. Add the flour and mix well. Add the milk and whisk until smooth. Cook and stir until thick and bubbly. Cook for 2 more minutes and add the cream cheese, paprika, cheddar cheese, mozzarella cheese, and turmeric. Cook over medium heat and stir until cheese is melted and smooth. Reduce heat to low and keep the cheese sauce heated over low heat. Don't forget to stir it. Coat the skillet with cooking spray and place over medium heat. Add the meat and cook until brown. Drain the fat and add in the taco seasoning. Cook for 5 minutes and stir until the water has evaporated. Arrange the tortilla on a serving plate, top with meat, cheese sauce, and the veggies. Serve.

Calories	Fat	Carbohydrates	Protein	Sodium

| 291 | 11g | 23g | 24g | 356mg |

Meatball Lasagna: Go Crazy with Beef and Pasta

Serves: 1

Ingredients:

- Lean ground beef [1 lb]
- Medium green sweet peppers stemmed, seeded and quartered [2 pcs]
- Shredded fresh basil or small fresh basil or oregano leaves
- Dried regular or whole-wheat lasagna noodles
- Snipped fresh flat-leaf parsley [2 tbsp]
- Salt [¼ tsp]
- Lasagna
- Soft whole-wheat breadcrumbs [¾ cup]
- Light ricotta cheese [¾ cup]
- Tomato sauce [3 tbsp]

- Shredded reduced-fat mozzarella cheese, divided [1½ cups]
- Ground black pepper [⅛ tsp]
- Chopped drained roasted red peppers [½ cup]
- Snipped fresh basil [¼ cup]
- Egg, lightly beaten [1 pc]
- Light or low-fat tomato-basil pasta sauce [1½ cups]
- Soft goat cheese (chèvre) or finely shredded Parmesan cheese [¼ cup]

Directions:

Preheat the oven to 350 deg. F and line the pan with foil. Add breadcrumbs, red peppers, egg, basil, parsley, tomato sauce, salt and pepper in a bowl. Add the ground beef and mix. Shape into 24 meatballs and place in a pan. Bake for 20 mins. Prepare the lasagna by increasing the oven temperature to 425 deg F. Line the sheet with foil and place the pepper quarters with the cut-sides down on the sheet. Roast for 20 minutes and do not cover. Wrap it in foil and let it cool for 20 mins. Peel the pepper quarters' skins and set aside. Reduce the oven temperature to 375 deg F. Cook the lasagna noodles based on packaging instructions and drain. Rinse with cold water and remove again then set aside. Add mozzarella, goat, and ricotta cheese in a bowl and mix. Spread half a cup of the pasta sauce on the baking dish. Layer two fo the cooked noodles on the plate. Add the meatballs on top and two more of cooked noodles. Top it with ricotta mixture. Add the peppers and the remaining cooked noodles. Spread the remaining sauce over it. Bake for 50 mins., without cover.

Uncover and sprinkle with remaining mozzarella. Baked unclever again for up to ten mins. Let it cool and serve.

Calories	Fat	Carbohydrates	Protein	Sodium
263	8g	22g	23g	468mg

Beef Kebabs: Grilled, Flavorful, and Delightful

Serves: 4-5

Ingredients:

Beef

- Garlic, minced [2 cloves]

- Lemon juice [1 tbsp]

- Finely shredded lemon peel [1 Tsp

- Olive oil [1 tbsp]

- Ground black pepper [1/4 Tsp

- Snipped fresh oregano [1 tbsp

- Ground cumin [1/2 tsp]

- Salt [1/2 tsp]

- Lean boneless beef top sirloin steak or top loin steak [1 lb]

Sauce

- Fresh oregano leaves [2 tbsp]

- Small shallots, peeled [2 pcs]

- Lemon juice [1 tbsp]

- Packed fresh Italian parsley leaves [1 1/3 cups]

- Olive oil [2 tbsp

- Salt [1/4 tsp]

- Crushed red pepper [1/8 tsp]

- Cider vinegar [2 tbsp]

- Garlic peeled [3 cloves]

Veggies

- Small boiling onions, peeled [8 oz]

- Medium green sweet pepper, cut into 1-1/2 inch pieces [1 pc]

- Whole button mushrooms [8 oz]

Directions:

Remove the fat from the meat and cut it into 1-inch size pieces. Place the meat in a plastic bag and set aside. Add lemon peel, olive oil, lemon juice, cumin, oregano, garlic, salt and pepper in a bowl and mix. Pour them over the meat and seal the bag. Marinate for 24 hours and turn the bag occasionally. Add oil, oregano, parsley, shallots, vinegar, garlic, salt, red pepper, and lemon juice in a blender and blend well. Cover and chill. Cook the onions in a saucepan with boiling water for three mins without lid. Drain and remove the meat from the marinade. Skewer the veggies and meat alternately and brush them with the marinade.

Place the kebabs on the grill, cover and cook for up to 12 minutes and making sure to turn them while grilling. Serve with sauce.

Calories	Fat	Carbohydrates	Protein	Sodium
281	16g	14g	23g	506mg

Beef and Veggie Ragout: A Must-Try French Classic Dish

Serves: 3-4

Ingredients:

- 14 oz can lower-sodium beef broth [2 pcs]
- Cherry tomatoes halved [2 cups]
- Minced garlic [4 cloves)
- Sliced fresh cremini or button mushrooms [3 cups
- Boneless beef chuck roast [1 ½ lbs]
- Port wine or dry sherry [1/2 cup
- Chopped onion [1 cup]
- Salt [1/2 Tsp
- Hot cooked noodles [4 cups]
- Ground black pepper [1/2 tsp]
- Quick-cooking tapioca crushed [1/4 cup]
- Sugar snap peas [4 cups]

Directions

Remove the fat from the meat and cut it into ¾-inch pieces. Lightly coat the skillet with cooking spray and place over medium-high heat. Add the meat and cook until meat is brown. Drain the fat off and set aside. Add the onion, salt, garlic, pepper, and mushrooms in the slow cooker. Sprinkle the tapioca and add the meat. Add the broth or the wine. Cover and cook on low heat for 8 to 10 hours. Add the sugar snap peas. Cover and let it cook for 5 minutes and add the cherry tomatoes. Serve over hot noodles.

Calories	Fat	Carbohydrates	Protein	Sodium
208	4g	19g	24g	401mg

Conclusion

Diabetes type 2, a disease that is known to have killed millions, is not as invincible as it may seem. I understand it takes more than just your physical health to suffer as soon as you get diagnosed. Some people may even suffer emotionally and psychologically as well. However, despite all the medications ready for you to take, all the recipes written in any book, and all the doctors and loved ones willing to help you through the way, nothing is possible unless you pick up the pieces and convince yourself that it is a fight you must face.

It all starts with you, your willingness and your commitment even after everything is said and done. Reversing diabetes takes patience and discipline. Condition yourself to that and be ready for a harsh ride. It's worth fighting for, I assure you.

After this book, you may feel like you need to find out more about your condition so feel free to observe yourself, ask professionals if needed, read books, and do not forget to record your progress and findings.

As for your food, don't let *what you put in your food* hinder you from enjoying it. Just because you have diabetes does not mean you are in for a life without sweetness. Explore the possibilities, and it will surely help you cope and eventually successfully reverse it. Thank you for purchasing this book!

Final Words

Thank you again for purchasing this book!

I really hope this book is able to help you.

The next step is for you to **join our email newsletter** to receive updates on any upcoming new book releases or promotions. You can sign-up for free and as a bonus, you will also receive our "*7 Fitness Mistakes You Don't Know You're Making*" book! This bonus book breaks down many of the most common fitness mistakes and will demystify many of the complexities and science of getting into shape. Having all this fitness knowledge and science organized into an actionable step-by-step book will help you get started in the right direction in your fitness journey! To join our free email newsletter and grab your free book, please visit the link and signup: **www.hmwpublishing.com/gift**

Finally, if you enjoyed this book, then I would like to ask you for a favor, would you be kind enough to leave a review for this book? It would be greatly appreciated!

Thank you and good luck in your journey!

About the Co-Author

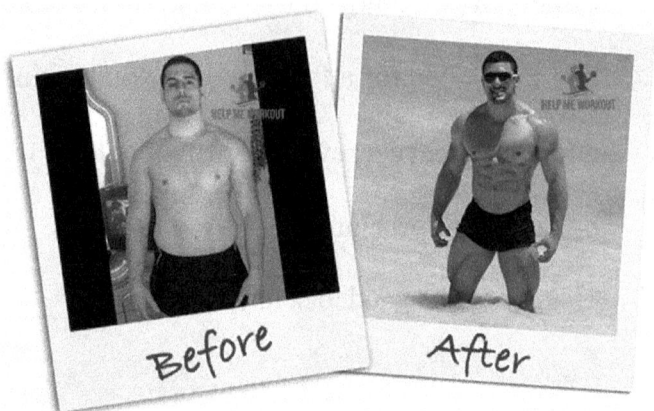

Before   After

My name is George Kaplo; I'm a certified personal trainer from Montreal, Canada. I'll start off by saying I'm not the biggest guy you will ever meet and this has never really been my goal. In fact, I started working out to overcome my biggest insecurity when I was younger, which was my self-confidence. This was due to my height measuring only 5 foot 5 inches (168cm), it pushed me down to attempt anything I ever wanted to achieve in life. You may be going through some challenges right now, or you may simply want to get fit, and I can certainly relate.

After a lot of work, studying and countless trial and errors. Some people began to notice how I was getting more fit and how I was starting to form a keen interest in the topic. This led many friends and new faces to come to me and ask me for fitness advice. At first, it seemed odd when people asked me to help them get in shape. But what kept me going is when they started to see changes in their own body and told me it's the first time that they saw real results! From there, more people kept coming to me, and it made me realize after so much reading and studying in this field that it did help me but it also allowed me to help others. I'm now a fully certified personal trainer and have trained numerous clients to date who have achieved amazing results.

Today, my brother Alex Kaplo (also a Certified Personal Trainer) and I own & operate this publishing venture, where we bring passionate and expert authors to write about health and fitness topics. We also run an online fitness website "HelpMeWorkout.com" and I would love to connect with by inviting you to visit the website on the following page and signing up to our e-mail newsletter (you will even get a free book).

Last but not least, if you are in the position I was once in and you want some guidance, don't hesitate and ask... I'll be there to help you out!

Your friend and coach,

George Kaplo

Certified Personal Trainer

Get another book for Free

I want to thank you for purchasing this book and offer you another book (just as long and valuable as this book), "Health & Fitness Mistakes You Don't Know You're Making", completely free.

Visit the link below to signup and receive it:

www.hmwpublishing.com/gift

In this book, I will break down the most common health & fitness mistakes, you are probably committing right now, and I will reveal how you can easily get in the best shape of your life!

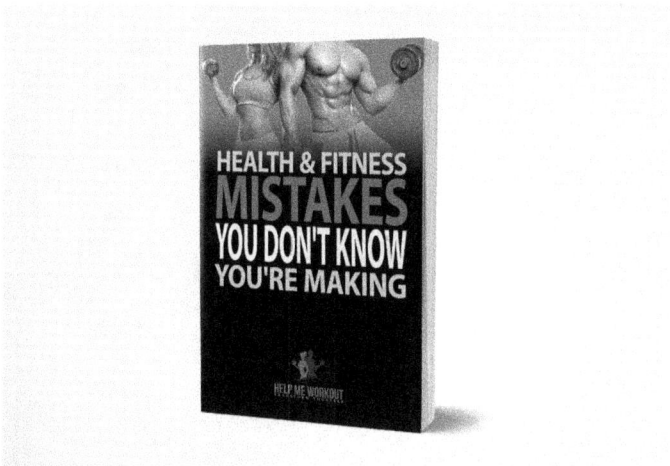

In addition to this valuable gift, you will also have an opportunity to get our new books for free, enter giveaways, and receive other valuable emails from me. Again, visit the link to sign up:

www.hmwpublishing.com/gift

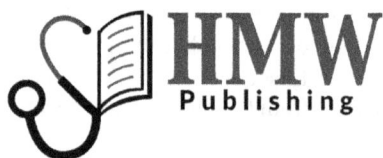

For more great books visit:

HMWPublishing.com

www.ingramcontent.com/pod-product-compliance
Lightning Source LLC
Chambersburg PA
CBHW060313030426
42336CB00011B/1033